I0484294

Evidence Synthesis

Number 111

Screening for Asymptomatic Carotid Artery Stenosis: A Systematic Review and Meta-Analysis for the U.S. Preventive Services Task Force

Prepared for:
Agency for Healthcare Research and Quality
U.S. Department of Health and Human Services
540 Gaither Road
Rockville, MD 20850
www.ahrq.gov

Contract No. HHSA-290-2012-00015-I, Task Order No. 2

Prepared by:
RTI International–University of North Carolina Evidence-based Practice Center
Research Triangle Park, NC

Investigators:
Daniel E. Jonas, MD, MPH
Cynthia Feltner, MD, MPH
Halle R. Amick, MSPH
Stacey Sheridan, MD, MPH
Zhi-Jie Zheng, MD, MPH, PhD
Daniel J. Watford, MD, MPH
Jamie L. Carter, MD, MPH
Cassandra J. Rowe, MPH
Russell Harris, MD, MPH

AHRQ Publication No. 13-05178-EF-1
July 2014

This report is based on research conducted by the RTI International–University of North Carolina Evidence-based Practice Center (EPC) under contract to the Agency for Healthcare Research and Quality (AHRQ), Rockville, MD (Contract No. HHSA-290-2012-00015-I, Task Order No. 2). The findings and conclusions in this document are those of the authors, who are responsible for its contents; the findings and conclusions do not necessarily represent the views of AHRQ. Therefore, no statement in this report should be construed as an official position of AHRQ or of the U.S. Department of Health and Human Services.

The information in this report is intended to help health care decisionmakers—patients and clinicians, health system leaders, and policymakers, among others—make well-informed decisions and thereby improve the quality of health care services. This report is not intended to be a substitute for the application of clinical judgment.

This report may be used, in whole or in part, as the basis for development of clinical practice guidelines and other quality enhancement tools, or as a basis for reimbursement and coverage policies. AHRQ or U.S. Department of Health and Human Services endorsement of such derivative products may not be stated or implied.

This document is in the public domain and may be used and reprinted without permission except those copyrighted materials that are clearly noted in the document. Further reproduction of those copyrighted materials is prohibited without the specific permission of copyright holders.

None of the investigators has any affiliations or financial involvement that conflicts with the material presented in this report.

Acknowledgments

The authors gratefully acknowledge the following individuals for their contributions to this project and deeply appreciate their considerable support, commitment, and contributions: Tracy Wolff, MD, MPH, AHRQ Medical Officer; Kirsten Bibbins-Domingo, PhD, MD, Jessica Herzstein, MD, MPH, and Michael LeFevre, MD, MSPH, U.S. Preventive Services Task Force leads; Evelyn Whitlock, MD, MPH, Kaiser Permanente Research Affiliates EPC director; Tracy Beil, MS, Kaiser Permanente Research Affiliates EPC; RTI International–University of North Carolina EPC staff: Carol Woodell, BSPH, project manager; Meera Viswanathan, PhD, EPC director; Christiane Voisin, MSLS, librarian; Laura Small, BA, editor; and Loraine Monroe, publications specialist.

Suggested Citation

Jonas DE, Feltner C, Amick HR, Sheridan S, Zheng ZJ, Watford DJ, et al. Screening for Asymptomatic Carotid Artery Stenosis: A Systematic Review and Meta-Analysis for the U.S. Preventive Services Task Force. Evidence Synthesis No. 111. AHRQ Publication No. 13-05178-EF-1. Rockville, MD: Agency for Healthcare Research and Quality; 2014.

Structured Abstract

Purpose: To evaluate the evidence on screening and treating asymptomatic adults for carotid artery stenosis (CAS) for the U.S. Preventive Services Task Force (USPSTF).

Data Sources: PubMed/MEDLINE, the Cochrane Library, EMBASE, and trial registries through September 2013; reference lists of published literature; MEDLINE searches for trials were updated through March 2014.

Study Selection: Two investigators independently selected studies reporting on asymptomatic adults with CAS, including randomized, controlled trials (RCTs) of screening for CAS; RCTs of carotid endarterectomy (CEA) or carotid angioplasty and stenting (CAAS) versus medical treatment; RCTs of medications versus placebo added to current standard medical therapy; multi-institution trials or cohort studies reporting harms; relevant systematic reviews; and studies that attempted to externally validate risk stratification tools.

Data Extraction: One reviewer extracted data and a second checked accuracy. Two independent reviewers assigned quality ratings using predefined criteria.

Data Synthesis: No RCTs compared screening with no screening, CAAS with medical treatment, or assessed intensification of medical therapy. Given the specificity of ultrasound (range 88% to 94% for CAS $\geq$50% to $\geq$70%), its use in low-prevalence populations would yield many false-positive results. Only one fair-quality study attempted external validation of a risk stratification tool to distinguish persons who are more likely to have CAS; the tool's discrimination was inadequate (c-statistic for $\geq$50% CAS, 0.60; 95% CI, 0.56 to 0.64). Our meta-analyses of RCTs comparing CEA with medical therapy found an absolute risk reduction of 5.5 percent (95% CI, 3.9 to 7.0) for any nonperioperative stroke over approximately 5 years. Meta-analyses for perioperative (30-day) stroke or death after CEA found rates of 2.4 percent (95% CI, 1.7 to 3.1) using all trials of CEA, regardless of the comparator; and 3.3 percent (95% CI, 2.7 to 3.9) using cohort studies (7 studies; n=17,474). Rates of perioperative stoke or death after CAAS were similar or slightly higher. Other important potential harms of CEA or CAAS include nonfatal perioperative myocardial infarction (approximately 0.8% rate after CEA), cranial nerve injury, pulmonary embolism, pneumonia, local hematoma requiring surgery, and psychological harms (e.g., anxiety or labeling). Externally validated, reliable risk stratification tools that can distinguish persons with asymptomatic CAS who have increased or decreased risk for ipsilateral stroke or harms after CEA or CAAS are not available.

Limitations: Medical therapy in trials varied and often lacked treatments that are now standard. For this reason, and because advances in medical therapy have reduced the rate of stroke in persons with asymptomatic CAS in recent decades, the true reduction of stroke or composite reduction of cardiovascular events is unknown. Trials utilized highly selected surgeons. No trials focused on a population identified by screening in primary care. Harms may be underreported.

Conclusion: Current evidence does not sufficiently establish incremental overall benefit of CEA, CAAS, or intensification of medical therapy beyond current standard medical therapy. Potential for overall benefit is limited by low prevalence in the general asymptomatic population and by harms from screening and treatment. Evidence is insufficient to allow reliable risk stratification.

Table of Contents

Figures

Figure 1. Analytic Framework

Figure 2. Summary of Evidence Search and Selection

Tables

Table 1. Studies Attempting to Externally Validate Risk Stratification Tools to Distinguish Persons Who Are More or Less Likely to Have CAS

Table 2. Characteristics of Included Randomized, Controlled Trials of CEA Compared With Medical Management for Asymptomatic CAS

Table 3. Main Results of Randomized, Controlled Trials of CEA Compared With Medical Management for Asymptomatic CAS

Table 4. Characteristics of Additional Studies Rated as Good or Fair Quality and Reporting Rates of Periprocedural Complications of CEA or CAAS for Adults With Asymptomatic CAS

Table 5. Results From Additional Studies Rated as Good or Fair Quality and Reporting Rates of Periprocedural Complications of CEA or CAAS for Adults With Asymptomatic CAS

Table 6. Projected 5-Year Outcomes of Screening 100,000 Asymptomatic Adults for CAS With Duplex Ultrasonography Followed by Confirmatory Testing With MRA

Appendixes

Appendix A. Summary of Recommendations From Other Groups

Appendix B. Detailed Methods

Appendix C. Excluded Studies

Appendix D. Quality Assessment of Included Studies

Appendix E. Additional Results

Appendix F. Results of Meta-Analyses

Chapter 1. Introduction

Scope and Purpose

The U.S. Preventive Services Task Force (USPSTF) last reviewed the evidence on screening for carotid artery stenosis (CAS) in 2007[1-3] and has commissioned an update of the evidence review to revisit its recommendation. The main purpose of this report is to systematically evaluate the current evidence on whether screening asymptomatic adults for CAS reduces the risk for fatal or nonfatal ipsilateral stroke and the evidence on harms associated with screening and interventions for CAS. Despite a D recommendation from the USPSTF in 2007,[3] many surgeries or interventions for asymptomatic CAS continue to be performed in the United States, and free screenings or those paid for out-of-pocket are offered in public locations across the country.[4]

The scope and methods of this report differ from earlier USPSTF reviews on this topic by 1) using systematic methods for all key questions (KQs) (the previous review reported using nonsystematic methods for three of its four questions),[2] 2) addressing new KQs about the availability of valid, reliable risk stratification tools to distinguish a person's likelihood for asymptomatic CAS and to distinguish risk for ipsilateral stroke caused by CAS or for harms from surgery or intervention in persons with asymptomatic CAS (recommendations of some groups state that screening might be considered for persons with multiple risk factors), 3) adding carotid angioplasty and stenting (CAAS) to the included interventions, 4) adding a question about the incremental benefit of medical therapy for asymptomatic CAS, and 5) conducting quantitative synthesis for many outcomes.

Condition Definition

Carotid artery stenosis refers to atherosclerotic narrowing of the extracranial carotid arteries. It typically refers to the internal carotid arteries or the common and internal carotid arteries. A "clinically important" degree of stenosis is defined as the percentage of stenosis that corresponds to a substantially increased risk for stroke. However, because stroke risk depends on more than just the degree of stenosis, it is difficult to set a lower limit on the range that defines potential clinical importance. The previous USPSTF recommendation considered clinically important CAS as stenosis ranging from 60 percent to 99 percent, but noted that minimum values of 50 percent and 70 percent have been used in some studies. Asymptomatic patients have no significant neurologic symptoms referable to the carotid artery and have not experienced a cerebrovascular event (i.e., a stroke or transient ischemic attack).

Prevalence and Burden

Stroke is a leading cause of death and disability in the United States. When considered separately from other cardiovascular diseases, stroke ranks as the fourth leading cause of death.[5] An estimated 7 million Americans age 20 years and older have had a stroke, and—of the approximately 800,000 strokes that occur in the United States per year—roughly 75 percent are first attacks.[6] Overall age-adjusted prevalence of stroke in 2010 was 2.6 percent.[7] Ischemic stroke accounts for nearly 90 percent of all strokes in the United States. Carotid artery stenosis is a risk factor for ischemic stroke. Because CAS progresses silently, a stroke can be the first indication of clinically significant stenosis. About 15 percent of ischemic strokes are caused by large artery atherothrombotic disease, which includes CAS.[8] Most ischemic strokes are not caused by CAS.

Stroke is among the leading causes of long-term disability in the United States.[9] Consequences of ischemic stroke include hemiparesis, aphasia, depression, and an array of limitations on activities of daily living.[10] The total cost of stroke in 2008 was $34.3 billion, and the cost of stroke from 2005 to 2050 is projected to exceed $2 trillion.[11]

The previous USPSTF review estimated the prevalence of 60 percent to 99 percent CAS to be about 1 percent in the general population of asymptomatic persons age 65 years and older. A recent systematic review and meta-analysis of cross-sectional and cohort studies estimated the pooled prevalence of asymptomatic CAS at 50 percent or greater to be 4.2 percent (95% CI, 3.1 to 5.7) and of asymptomatic CAS at 70 percent or greater to be 1.7 percent (95% CI, 0.7 to 3.9).[12] Both age and sex influenced the prevalence estimates. For adults younger than age 70 years, the pooled prevalence estimates for CAS at 50 percent or greater were 2.2 percent for women and 4.8 percent for men; for persons age 70 years or older, estimates were 6.9 percent and 12.5 percent, respectively.[12] Rates reported in the meta-analysis included complete occlusion (i.e., 100% CAS), and the included studies were quite heterogeneous with respect to demographics, methods of ascertaining stenosis, and quality. Very few studies sampled U.S. general populations, and just four studies, all from outside the United States, contributed data for the analysis of CAS at 70 percent or greater.

The best available data from large U.S.-based studies of the general population (Cardiovascular Health Study) were published in the 1990s and enrolled adults ages 65 and older.[14] Data published in 1992 showed prevalence of 75 to 99 percent CAS was 1.07 percent (31/2,906) for women and 1.22 percent (27/2,210) for men.[13] Rates for 75 to 100 percent CAS were 1.14 percent and 2.26 percent, respectively. Data published in 1998 suggest an overall prevalence of 70 to 99 percent CAS to be 0.5 percent, based on prevalence of peak systolic velocity greater than or equal to 2.5 m/s.[14]

Etiology and Natural History

Carotid artery narrowing is most commonly caused by the buildup of fat, cholesterol, calcium, and other fibrous substances (commonly known as "plaque") in the arteries over time. Carotid artery stenosis can restrict blood flow to the brain in several ways. This can occur as a result of artery-to-artery embolism of atherosclerotic plaque fragments or thrombotic occlusion of the internal carotid artery. Common contributors to CAS include hypertension, diabetes, smoking, and high cholesterol (particularly a high level of low-density lipoproteins [LDL]).

Several studies have attempted to estimate the rate of progression of asymptomatic CAS and to predict neurologic events resulting from CAS.[14-19] Many studies have small samples and are unlikely to be representative of the general asymptomatic population. The potential development of collaterals complicates determining a direct relationship between CAS and resulting stroke; persons with complete occlusion may or may not have a stroke.

The best available data from large U.S.-based studies of the general population (Cardiovascular Health Study) showed a 5 percent 5-year risk for fatal or nonfatal ipsilateral stroke for CAS at 70 percent or greater (n=5,441).[14] Smaller studies from single centers in New York (n=425, all asymptomatic) and Illinois (n=142/272 asymptomatic) followed patients with 50 to 79 percent CAS and reported new ipsilateral strokes in 3.8 percent over a mean followup of approximately 3.2 years[19] or mean annual stroke rates of 2 percent over a mean followup of approximately 3.7 years.[17] Little data on followup beyond 5 years exist; one Canadian cohort study using the subgroup that completed at least 5 years of followup (106 persons from an initial cohort of 500) reported 10- and 15-year rates of 9.3 percent and 16.6 percent, respectively, for patients with 50 to 99 percent CAS.[20] Thus, the available data indicate that the vast majority of patients with asymptomatic CAS will not have a stroke caused by their CAS within 5 or 10 years.

In general, risk factors for ischemic stroke are thought to include age greater than 65 years, male sex, hypertension, heart disease, smoking or tobacco use, high blood cholesterol and other lipids, physical inactivity, and diabetes mellitus.[21] The previous review for the USPSTF indicated that there are no validated risk stratification tools to discriminate persons with asymptomatic CAS who are at high risk for stroke compared with persons at low risk, although a specific, systematic search for these tools was not conducted.[1]

Rationale for Screening and Screening Strategies

Stroke remains a leading cause of death and disability in the United States. In theory, screening might be able to identify asymptomatic CAS for possible treatment before it causes health problems. The most common screening test for CAS is carotid duplex ultrasonography, with or without confirmatory testing using digital subtraction angiography (the gold standard). Because confirmatory testing using digital subtraction angiography can have complications such as stroke, it is rarely used in routine clinical practice. Other potential screening or confirmatory tests include computed tomography angiography (CTA) and magnetic resonance angiography (MRA).

Treatment Approaches

Potential therapeutic options for asymptomatic CAS include carotid endarterectomy (CEA) and medical therapy, CAAS and medical therapy, or medical therapy alone. In CEA, a surgeon clamps the internal, common, and external carotid arteries, opens the lumen of the internal carotid artery, and removes the plaque. Then, the artery and overlying layers are closed. Many surgeons use a shunt to ensure blood supply to the brain during the procedure. The procedure may be performed under general or local anesthesia.

In CAAS, an interventionist typically accesses the vasculature by inserting a catheter into the femoral artery, up to the aortic arch, and then up the carotid artery. Then, the catheter dilates a balloon to open the artery and inserts a stent to hold it open.

Current standard medical therapy to reduce stroke risk has evolved, and it now includes: use of 3-hydroxy-3-methylglutaryl-coenzyme (HMG-CoA) reductase inhibitors (i.e., statins); control of blood pressure with antihypertensives (including newer classes of medications, such as ACE inhibitors); glycemic control for persons with diabetes; and use of antiplatelet drugs for vascular diseases and risk reduction. Statin therapy, in particular, is thought to have beneficial effects on carotid plaque morphology and the inflammatory response.[22] Standard medical practice has evolved as the evidence on screening for CAS has developed. In general, medical therapy in 2014 is more aggressive in reaching lower blood pressure and LDL targets than it was 10 years ago. Thus, the risk for stroke has decreased with improvements in medical therapy. Lifestyle modifications (smoking cessation, increased physical activity, improved diet) may also help prevent carotid stenosis–related stroke.[21]

Decisions between various treatment approaches may involve tradeoffs between benefits and risks. For example, surgery or intervention may introduce significant short-term risks of stroke, death, or myocardial infarction (MI) (as harms of surgery or intervention) in exchange for long-term reduction in risks of stroke or death.

Current Clinical Practice in the United States

Large studies involving data from Medicare claims show significant geographic variation in the rates of CEA and, to a lesser extent, carotid stenting; however, these studies may be limited by their ability to collect detailed information on symptom status. One cohort study of Medicare beneficiaries reported rates of 2.8 CEAs per 1,000 beneficiaries and 0.3 CAASs per 1,000 beneficiaries.[23] Substantial geographic variation existed, with a nearly nine-fold difference between the highest rate and lowest rates of CEAs across hospital referral regions.[23] This same study also found considerable variation in the type of diagnostic imaging performed before carotid revascularization.

Accurate information on current rates of CEA and carotid stenting for asymptomatic patients in the general population is difficult to obtain because detailed data on symptom status may not reside in large registries (e.g., Medicare claims data). One study of Medicare beneficiaries in New York state linked Medicare claims with medical records (including detailed information on symptom status) and found that about three-quarters (72.3%) of patients who underwent CEA in 2007 were asymptomatic.[24] A smaller 2012 study conducted in four urban hospitals found that 63 percent of CEAs performed within a 2-year period were for asymptomatic patients.[25] Evidence also reveals variation in the use of procedures by physician specialty. A recent analysis of carotid stenting in Medicare beneficiaries found that cardiologists perform half of the procedures and significant differences were noted in the characteristics of patients treated by cardiologists compared with other specialists.[26] Population-based utilization rates for carotid stenting were significantly higher in hospital referral regions where cardiologists performed most procedures compared with regions where other specialists primarily performed the procedures. Although detailed symptom status was not available, patients treated by cardiologists had fewer neurologic conditions, including less evidence of recent acute stroke or transient ischemic attack, in the 180 days prior to stenting. More than 50 percent of patients treated by cardiologists also underwent cardiac catheterization prior to carotid stenting and had carotid and cerebral angiography performed simultaneously, suggesting the possibility that routine case findings of severe CAS by cardiologists during diagnostic angiography influenced patient selection.[26]

Previous USPSTF Recommendation

In 2007, the USPSTF recommended that providers should not screen for asymptomatic CAS in the general adult population (D recommendation).[3] Recommendations from other groups similarly discourage screening for the general population. However, several guidelines suggest that screening for asymptomatic CAS may be appropriate for patients thought to be at high risk (Appendix A).

Chapter 2. Methods

Key Questions and Analytic Framework

The investigators, USPSTF members, and Agency for Healthcare Research and Quality (AHRQ) Medical Officers developed the scope and KQs for this review. The analytic framework illustrates the KQs that guided the review (Figure 1).

Key Questions

1. Is there direct evidence that screening adults with duplex ultrasonography, CTA, and/or MRA for asymptomatic CAS reduces fatal or nonfatal ipsilateral stroke?
    a. Is there direct evidence for persons at decreased risk?
    b. Is there direct evidence for persons at average risk?
    c. Is there direct evidence for persons at increased risk?
    d. Does the evidence differ for subgroups defined by age, sex, race, or ethnicity?
2. Are externally validated, reliable risk stratification tools available that distinguish persons who are more or less likely to have CAS (defined as 60% to 99% stenosis)?
3a. What is the accuracy and reliability of screening with duplex ultrasonography, used alone or followed by CTA or MRA, to detect potentially clinically important CAS (defined as 60% to 99% stenosis)?
3b. Do the accuracy and reliability differ for subgroups defined by age, sex, race, or ethnicity?
4a. Are externally validated, reliable risk stratification tools available that distinguish persons with asymptomatic CAS (defined as 60% to 99% stenosis) who are at decreased or increased risk for ipsilateral stroke caused by CAS?
4b. Are externally validated, reliable risk stratification tools available that distinguish persons with asymptomatic CAS who are at decreased or increased risk for harms from CEA or CAAS?
5. For persons with asymptomatic CAS (defined as 60% to 99% stenosis), does intervention with carotid endarterectomy (CEA) or carotid angioplasty and stenting (CAAS) provide incremental benefit beyond current standard medical therapy for reduction of fatal or nonfatal ipsilateral stroke?
    a. Is there incremental benefit for persons at decreased risk for ipsilateral stroke caused by CAS?
    b. Is there incremental benefit for persons at average risk for ipsilateral stroke caused by CAS?
    c. Is there incremental benefit for persons at increased risk for ipsilateral stroke caused by CAS?
    d. Does the evidence differ for subgroups defined by age, sex, race, or ethnicity?
6. For persons with asymptomatic CAS (defined as 60% to 99% stenosis), does the addition of medications (e.g., aspirin, statins) provide incremental benefit beyond current standard medical therapy that includes treatment of traditional risk factors (e.g., hypertension, hypercholesterolemia) for reduction of fatal or nonfatal ipsilateral stroke?

a. Is there incremental benefit for persons at decreased risk for ipsilateral stroke caused by CAS?
b. Is there incremental benefit for persons at average risk for ipsilateral stroke caused by CAS?
c. Is there incremental benefit for persons at increased risk for ipsilateral stroke caused by CAS?
d. Does the evidence differ for subgroups defined by age, sex, race, or ethnicity?

7a. What are the harms associated with screening or confirmatory testing for asymptomatic CAS?

7b. Do the harms differ for subgroups defined by age, sex, race, or ethnicity?

7c. Do the harms differ for subgroups defined by comorbidities?

8a. What are the harms associated with CEA or CAAS for the treatment of asymptomatic CAS?

8b. Do the harms differ for subgroups defined by age, sex, race, or ethnicity?

8c. Do the harms differ for subgroups defined by comorbidities?

Contextual Questions

We addressed the following contextual question: What is the accuracy and reliability of auscultation for carotid bruit to detect potentially clinically important CAS (60% to 99% stenosis)?

Data Sources and Searches

We searched PubMed/MEDLINE, the Cochrane Library, and EMBASE for English-language articles published through September 2013. We conducted a targeted update search for trials published through March 31, 2014, limited to MEDLINE. We used Medical Subject Headings (MeSH) as search terms when available and keywords when appropriate, focusing on terms to describe relevant populations, screening tests, interventions, outcomes, and study designs. Complete search terms and limits are listed in Appendix B. We conducted targeted searches for unpublished literature by searching ClinicalTrials.gov, the Cochrane Stroke Group Trials Registry, and the World Health Organization International Clinical Trials Registry Platform (WHO ICTRP). To supplement electronic searches, we reviewed the reference lists of pertinent review articles and studies that met our inclusion criteria and added all previously unidentified relevant articles. We reviewed all literature suggested by peer reviewers or public comment respondents and, if appropriate, incorporated it into the final review.

Study Selection

We developed inclusion and exclusion criteria for populations, interventions, comparators, outcomes, timing, settings, and study designs[27] (Appendix B Table 1). We included studies focused on asymptomatic adults with CAS, but also included studies that enrolled both symptomatic and asymptomatic subjects if the asymptomatic group was analyzed separately. For the population of interest, we did not rigidly consider persons with 60 to 99 percent CAS as a single homogeneous cohort. Rather, we included studies enrolling subjects that went beyond that degree of CAS (e.g., VACS [Veterans Affairs Cooperative Study] allowed enrollment of persons with 50% to 99% CAS), and we evaluated the available evidence for subgroups in that cohort. For example, we evaluated evidence for persons with 80 to 99 percent CAS, if available. For KQ 1, we searched for randomized, controlled trials (RCTs) comparing screened with nonscreened groups. For KQ 2, we included studies that developed risk stratification tools, and then validated the tools using an external population. For KQ 3, we focused on systematic reviews, but also included primary studies that were published after the included systematic reviews. For KQ 4, we searched for cohort studies that developed risk stratification tools, and then validated the tools using an external population. We required studies to follow a cohort of adults with asymptomatic CAS to develop a tool predicting risk for ipsilateral stroke (KQ 4a) or periprocedural harms (KQ 4b). For both KQ 2 and KQ 4, we required that risk stratification tools (or "risk prediction tools") combined multiple variables and allowed us to calculate risk for individual patients. Risk stratification tools may include clinical factors (e.g., age, diabetes) and anatomic or imaging predictors (e.g., plaque area or morphology, silent embolic events, contralateral disease). For KQ 5, we included systematic reviews and RCTs comparing CEA or CAAS with medical treatment. For KQ 6, we searched for systematic reviews and RCTs that compared the addition of one or more medications to current standard medical therapy (including treatment of traditional risk factors) with the addition of placebo to current standard medical therapy (including treatment of traditional risk factors). For KQs 7 and 8, we included systematic reviews, multi-institution trials, or cohort studies (including registries) reporting rates of relevant harms.

Two investigators independently reviewed titles and abstracts; those marked for potential inclusion by either reviewer were retrieved for evaluation of the full text. Then, two investigators independently reviewed the full texts to determine final inclusion or exclusion. Disagreements were resolved by an experienced team member.

Quality Assessment and Data Abstraction

We extracted pertinent information from each article, including information about the methods, populations, interventions, comparators, outcomes, timing, settings, and study designs. A second team member reviewed all data extractions for completeness and accuracy.

We assessed the quality of studies as good, fair, or poor using predefined criteria (Appendix D).[28] Two independent reviewers assigned quality ratings for each study. Disagreements were resolved by discussion with an experienced team member.

Data Synthesis and Analysis

We qualitatively synthesized findings for each key question by summarizing the characteristics and results of included studies in tabular or narrative format. To determine whether meta-analyses were appropriate, we assessed the clinical and methodological heterogeneity of the studies following established guidance.[29] We qualitatively assessed the populations, interventions, comparators, outcomes, and study designs of the included studies, looking for similarities and differences.

We conducted quantitative synthesis of RCTs comparing CEA with medical therapy using meta-analyses of relevant outcomes reported by multiple studies. We used random-effects models (DerSimonian and Laird) using the inverse-variance weighted method to estimate pooled effects.[30] We calculated risk differences between groups to reflect the absolute difference between CEA and medical therapy. We calculated rates using the number of all randomized patients as the denominator to reflect a true intention-to-treat analysis. For ACAS (Asymptomatic Carotid Atherosclerosis Study), we used the actual observed numbers of events (reported for median followup of 2.7 years) rather than the projected/estimated 5-year rates.[31] For ACST, we used complete data from the 10-year publication.[32]

We conducted quantitative synthesis of composite outcomes that included key benefits and harms and that were the primary outcomes in ACAS and ACST (Asymptomatic Carotid Surgery Trial): 1) perioperative stroke or death (within 30 days) and subsequent ipsilateral stroke and 2) perioperative stroke or death (within 30 days) and any subsequent stroke. We also conducted quantitative synthesis for the following outcomes assessing potential benefits and harms: all-cause mortality, any stroke or death, ipsilateral nonperioperative stroke (i.e., occurring after the perioperative period), any nonperioperative stroke, perioperative stroke or death, and perioperative myocardial infarction.

To allow some comparison of rates of perioperative harms reported in RCTs with those from sources that may be more representative of real-world clinical practice, we conducted meta-analyses of noncomparative cohort studies (including registries) reporting perioperative (30-day) stroke or death rates. We also conducted meta-analyses of perioperative stroke or death rates reported in trials involving CEA or CAAS, regardless of the comparator. We analyzed rates for CEA and CAAS separately. When articles did not report 95 percent confidence intervals for rates of perioperative stroke or death, we calculated 95 percent confidence intervals using the Wilson method.[33] Random-effects models were used to estimate pooled event rates.

The chi-squared statistic and the I^2 statistic (the proportion of variation in study estimates due to heterogeneity) were calculated to assess statistical heterogeneity in effects between studies.[34,35] An I^2 from 0 to 40 percent might not be important, 30 percent to 60 percent may represent moderate heterogeneity, 50 percent to 90 percent may represent substantial heterogeneity, and 75 percent or greater represents considerable heterogeneity.[36] The importance of the observed value of I^2 depends on the magnitude and direction of effects and on the strength of evidence for heterogeneity (e.g., p value from the chi-squared test or a confidence interval for I^2).

We conducted several types of sensitivity analyses. First, because DerSimonian and Laird random-effects models may not perform well for small meta-analyses (when few studies are included), we conducted sensitivity analyses using profile likelihood random-effects methods.[37-40] Results for profile likelihood meta-analyses were essentially the same as for our main analyses, with some minor variation in width of confidence intervals. Therefore, the results are only provided in the appendix of meta-analyses (Appendix F), and are not discussed in the text. Next, we did not include studies rated as poor quality in any main analyses, but did include them in sensitivity analyses. Finally, for our meta-analyses of RCTs comparing CEA with medical therapy that included perioperative stroke or death outcomes, we conducted sensitivity analyses including angiogram-related stroke or death occurring prior to surgery (both ACAS and VACS required preoperative confirmatory angiograms) to reflect the harms of the screening cascade if confirmatory angiograms are used. Such events were not included in our main analyses. All quantitative analyses were conducted using Stata® version 11.1 (StataCorp LP, College Station, TX).

Expert Review and Public Comment

A draft report was reviewed by content experts, USPSTF members, and AHRQ Medical Officers, and was revised based on comments.

USPSTF Involvement

This review was funded by AHRQ. Staff of AHRQ and members of the USPSTF participated in developing the scope of the work and reviewed draft manuscripts, but the authors are solely responsible for the content.

Chapter 3. Results

Literature Search

Of the 3,938 unique records identified, we assessed 477 full texts for eligibility (Figure 2). After excluding 399 articles (see Appendix C), we included 78 published articles reporting on 56 studies. Of the included studies (articles), three (12) were RCTs comparing CEA with medical management, eight (10) were systematic reviews, one (3) assessed risk stratification tools for KQ 2, three (4) were primary studies assessing accuracy or reliability of screening for KQ 3, and 41 (49) were multi-institution studies reporting rates of relevant harms for KQs 7 or 8. We rated the quality of 21 studies as poor. Details are provided under the relevant KQs in this chapter, and full quality assessments are provided in Appendix D.

Results of Included Studies

Key Question 1. Direct Evidence That Screening for Asymptomatic CAS Reduces Fatal or Nonfatal Ipsilateral Stroke

We found no eligible studies that addressed this question.

Key Question 2. Externally Validated, Reliable Risk Stratification Tools to Distinguish Persons Who Are More or Less Likely to Have CAS

We found one study[41] that attempted to externally validate two previously developed tools for predicting the likelihood of significant CAS in asymptomatic general populations (Table 1). One of the tools[42] assigned one point each for the presence of several risk factors (existing coronary artery disease [CAD], smoking, hypertension, and high cholesterol) to predict the likelihood of CAS at 50 percent or greater. The other tool[43] assigned weighted points for each of an overlapping set of risk factors (existing CAD = 2 points, smoking = 1 point, high cholesterol = 1 point, age greater than 65 years = 4 points) to predict the likelihood of CAS at 60 percent or greater. The publication that attempted to externally validate both tools used a cohort of 5,449 persons from the Cardiovascular Health Study.[41] Mean age in this cohort was 72 years. Forty-two percent of the cohort were male, and 82 percent were white. Eight percent reported known CAD.

The attempts to externally validate the two risk prediction tools provided limited information regarding predictive validity. We rated the external validation of the tool that assigned weighted points as poor quality, mainly because its prediction of CAS risk levels and its testing of an altered scoring system that differed from those used in the derivation cohort. In the best-quality attempted external validation,[41,42] persons with the highest risk score were more likely to have CAS at 50 percent or greater than persons with lower risk scores (4 points = 21%, 3 points = 8%, 2 points = 5%, 1 point = 3%, and 0 points = 3%). The likelihood of a positive test was higher in persons with CAS at 50 percent or greater than in persons with CAS less than 50 percent (+LR 6 for a score of 4). However, the tool's overall discrimination (i.e., its ability to correctly assign persons with CAS at 50 percent or greater to a higher score than persons with lesser CAS) was little better than chance (c-statistic, 0.60 [95% CI, 0.56 to 0.64]). A c-statistic less than 0.70 is thought to indicate inadequate discrimination.[44,45] Calibration, often assessed by plotting the predicted risk versus the observed event rate,[44] was not reported.

Key Question 3. Accuracy and Reliability of Duplex Ultrasonography

We included three meta-analyses[46-48] and three primary studies[49-52] assessing the accuracy and/or reliability of duplex ultrasonography to detect CAS. Two of the three primary studies were rated as poor quality. The most recent good-quality meta-analysis[46] included studies published from 1966 to 2003 and assessed the accuracy of duplex ultrasonography using digital subtraction angiography as the reference standard. For detecting CAS at 50 percent or greater, the authors reported a sensitivity of 98 percent (95% CI, 97 to 100) and a specificity of 88 percent (95% CI, 76 to 100). For detecting CAS at 70 percent or greater, the sensitivity and specificity were 90 percent (95% CI, 84 to 94) and 94 percent (95% CI, 88 to 97), respectively. The 2007 evidence report for the USPSTF[1] used information from the meta-analysis to estimate the sensitivity and specificity for detecting stenosis at 60 percent or greater as 94 percent and 92 percent, respectively. The findings of the other meta-analyses and the primary studies are generally consistent with these results, however, specificities from two of the primary studies were lower. Results of all included studies are provided in Appendix E. The other meta-analyses were either relatively outdated (published in 1995[48]) or only included studies published during a selected time period (1993 to 2001[47]). None of the included studies reported whether (or what proportion of) asymptomatic patients were included.

The reliability of duplex ultrasonography to detect potentially clinically important CAS is limited. The good-quality meta-analysis reported wide variation in measurement properties between laboratories, with clinically important variation in the magnitude of the variation.[46] Potential sources of measurement heterogeneity include differences in patients, study designs, equipment, techniques, or training.[46] For example, different methods of classification will diagnose CAS at different degrees. The European Carotid Surgery Trial (ECST) method compares the diameter of the residual lumen at the site of the maximal luminal narrowing with the estimated normal lumen at the same site, however, the NASCET (the North American Symptomatic Carotid Endarterectomy Trial) method compares the maximal luminal narrowing diameter with the normal diameter of the artery distal to the stenosis. The ECST method generally yields a higher degree of CAS than the NASCET method and with clinically important differences between the two methods. Two analyses[53,54] found that the ECST method resulted in between 12[54] and 51[53] percent more stenoses classified as 70 to 99 percent, than with the NASCET method. Sabeti et al.[51] studied 1,006 carotid arteries and found poor agreement between readers for the differentiation of stenoses less than 70 percent (45% agreement; kappa 0.26 [95% CI, 0.23 to 0.29]), but excellent agreement for stenosis at 70 percent or greater (96% agreement; kappa 0.85 [95% CI, 0.83 to 0.87]). Hwang et al. reported little variability in sensitivity, but significant differences in specificity when they compared the ECST with the NASCET method.[52] Results of duplex ultrasonography screening can also vary based on the type of scanner,[55] velocity cutpoints and/or ratios used,[56] Doppler angle employed,[50,57] and inherent variability between facilities and observers.[58,59]

We did not find any eligible studies that directly addressed whether accuracy and reliability differ for subgroups defined by age, sex, race, or ethnicity.

Key Question 4. Externally Validated, Reliable Risk Stratification Tools to Distinguish Persons With Asymptomatic CAS Who Are at Decreased or Increased Risk for Stroke Caused by CAS or Decreased or Increased Risk for Harms From CEA or CAAS

We found no eligible studies that addressed this question. Some publications reported risk stratification tools to predict who is at decreased or increased risk for complications from CEA or CAAS (see the Discussion section), but those tools have not been externally validated.[60-66] We found no studies that reported risk stratification tools to predict who is at decreased or increased risk for ipsilateral stroke or death caused by CAS.

Key Question 5. Incremental Benefit of CEA or CAAS Beyond Current Standard Medical Therapy for Reduction of Fatal or Nonfatal Ipsilateral Stroke

We included three RCTs described in 12 publications[31,32,67-76] comparing CEA with medical therapy and three good- or fair-quality systematic reviews described in five publications.[1,2,77-79] Two systematic reviews were rated as poor quality.[80,81] We found no eligible studies that compared CAAS with medical therapy and no studies that compared CEA with current standard medical therapy.

Trial Characteristics

Table 2 summarizes the characteristics of the RCTs. A total of 5,226 patients were enrolled. ACAS and VACS were conducted in North America, and ACST involved 30 countries, primarily in Europe. None of the trials focused on a population identified by screening in primary care. Mean age of subjects was 65 to 68 years. The vast majority (87% to 95%) of subjects were white in the two North American trials (data not reported for ACST). Two thirds of enrolled subjects (ACAS and ACST) or more (100% in VACS) were men.

Although subjects were deemed asymptomatic with relation to the ipsilateral carotid artery, 20 to 24 percent had a history of prior contralateral CEA and 25 to 32 percent had a history of contralateral transient ischemic attack or stroke in trials reporting baseline data for these characteristics. Requirements for asymptomatic status differed slightly across the trials. For example, ACST enrolled subjects with no transient ischemic attack or stroke attributable to the ipsilateral artery for the past 6 months; ACAS enrolled persons with no history of cerebrovascular events in the distribution of the ipsilateral carotid artery or the vertebrobasilar system, and no symptoms referable to the contralateral artery for the past 45 days. For inclusion, subjects were required to have at least 50 percent (VACS) or at least 60 percent (ACAS and ACST) CAS.

Medical therapy varied across trials and was often not clearly defined or standardized. All subjects received aspirin in ACAS and VACS. ACAS also included a risk factor discussion and modification at randomization, subsequent interviews, and telephone followup. ACST left medical therapy to the discretion of clinicians, reporting that it usually included antiplatelet and antihypertensive therapy and, in later years of the trial, lipid-lowering therapy.

Surgeons with a history of low complication rates were selected for the three trials. They submitted records of their last 50 cases (ACAS and ACST) or previous 24 months of experience with CEA (VACS) and were selected based on demonstrated acceptability of morbidity and mortality (either based on review by a committee or a morbidity and mortality rate less than 3%). In addition, ACAS and ACST trial protocols included stipulations to prevent further enrollment by surgeons or institutions that showed unacceptably high morbidity or mortality during the trial.

Trial Results

Table 3 summarizes the main results of the three trials, and Appendix F includes complete results of our meta-analyses. Risk differences represent absolute differences over approximately 5 years.

Perioperative stroke or death or subsequent ipsilateral stroke. Our meta-analyses found that 2.0 percent fewer subjects treated with CEA had perioperative stroke or death or subsequent ipsilateral stroke compared with subjects in medical therapy groups (risk difference [RD], -0.020 [95% CI, -0.033 to -0.007]).

Perioperative stroke or death or any subsequent stroke. Our meta-analyses found that 3.5 percent fewer subjects treated with CEA had perioperative stroke or death or any subsequent stroke compared with subjects in medical therapy groups (RD, -0.035 [95% CI, -0.051 to -0.018]).

All-cause mortality. Our meta-analyses found no difference between CEA and medical therapy (RD, 0.01 [95% CI, -0.02 to 0.03]).

Any stroke or death. Our meta-analyses found that 2.7 percent fewer subjects treated with CEA had any stroke or death compared with subjects in medical therapy groups (RD, -0.027 [95% CI, -0.051 to -0.003]).

Ipsilateral stroke (nonperioperative). Our meta-analyses found that 4.1 percent fewer subjects treated with CEA had ipsilateral stroke compared with subjects in medical therapy groups (RD, -0.041 [95% CI, -0.054 to -0.027]), not including the perioperative period.

Any nonperioperative stroke. Our meta-analyses found that 5.5 percent fewer subjects treated with CEA had any stroke after the perioperative period compared with subjects in medical therapy groups (RD, -0.055 [95% CI, -0.070 to -0.039]).

Quality of life and functional status. None of the included trials assessed quality of life using validated instruments (e.g., SF-36), but two reported some information about stroke severity. In ACST, more than half (57.8% or 166/287) of nonperioperative strokes were disabling or fatal and the proportional reduction in disabling or fatal stroke (RR, 0.61 [95% CI, 0.41 to 0.92]) was similar to that for any stroke (RR, 0.54 [95% CI, 0.43 to 0.68]).[32] In VACS, mean stroke severity scores were 3.6 and 4.1 for the CEA and medical therapy groups, respectively (range not reported, p value reported as not statistically significant), indicating minor impairment on average (1 to 11 scale, with scores of 1 to 3 indicating no impairment, score of 4 indicating minor impairment, and scores of 5 or greater indicating major impairment in at least one domain of functioning).[73]

Persons at decreased, average, or increased risk for ipsilateral stroke. As described in KQ 4, we did not find any externally validated, reliable risk stratification tools to distinguish persons with asymptomatic CAS who are at decreased or increased risk for stroke caused by CAS. Therefore, evidence does not allow reliable determination of whether the potential benefits of CEA or CAAS differ for persons at decreased, average, and increased risk for ipsilateral stroke caused by CAS.

Age, sex, race, and ethnicity. None of the trials reported subgroup information by race or ethnicity. The ACAS and ACST provided subgroup analyses for some outcomes by sex and age. In ACAS, the estimated 5-year rate of perioperative stroke or death and subsequent ipsilateral stroke showed a statistically significant reduction for men (RRR, 66% [95% CI, 36 to 82]), but not for women (17% [95% CI, -96 to 65]). Subgroup analyses by age for the same outcome showed a significant reduction for persons younger than age 68 years (RRR, 60% [95% CI, 11 to 82]), but not for persons age 68 years and older (43% [95% CI, -7 to 70]). Subgroup analyses by percent CAS (60% to 69.9%, 70% to 79.9%, and 80% to 99.9%) found no statistically significant gradation in reduction, but sample sizes were small.

In ACST, reduction in first nonperioperative stroke was statistically significant for both sex subgroups (men RR, 0.52 [95% CI, 0.36 to 0.75]; women RR, 0.57 [95% CI, 0.34 to 0.97]). For subgroups defined by age, reduction in the first nonperioperative stroke was significant for persons younger than age 75 years, but not for persons age 75 and older (age <65 years RR, 0.46 [95% CI, 0.26 to 0.82]; age 65 to 74 years RR, 0.48 [95% CI, 0.31 to 0.75]; age ≥75 years RR, 0.81 [95% CI, 0.43 to 1.51]). Subgroup analyses by percent CAS (<70%, 70% to 79%, 80% to 89%, 90% to 99%) found similar point estimates for patients with varying degrees of CAS.

Systematic Reviews

Two of the three reviews included good- or fair-quality systematic reviews comparing CEA with medical management were conducted prior to the most recent ACST publication,[32] and thus had preliminary ACST data; these reviews were the last review for the USPSTF[2] and a review on CEA for asymptomatic CAS from the Cochrane Collaboration.[77] The third review compared management strategies for asymptomatic CAS and included a meta-regression to evaluate the effect of time (to reflect improvements in medical therapy) on incidence rates of stroke.[78] The investigators found that the incidence rate of ipsilateral stroke was lower in studies that completed recruitment from 2000 to 2010 than in studies that completed recruitment in earlier years (1.13% vs. 2.38% per year; p<0.001).[78]

Key Question 6. Incremental Benefit of Additional Medications Beyond Current Standard Medical Therapy

We found no eligible studies that addressed this question.

Key Question 7. Harms Associated With Screening or Confirmatory Testing

The potential harms of screening or confirmatory testing for asymptomatic CAS include harms associated with false-positive screening tests (e.g., anxiety, labeling) and harms of any confirmatory workup, such as angiography. We found no studies on anxiety or labeling in persons with false-positive results. Two RCTs reported strokes after angiography. In ACAS,[31] 5 of 414 patients (1.2%) who underwent angiograms developed strokes; one of these five patients died subsequently. In VACS,[73] 3 of 714 patients (0.4%) had nonfatal strokes following angiography. Evidence was insufficient to determine whether the harms differ for subgroups defined by age, sex, race, ethnicity, or comorbidities.

Key Question 8. Harms Associated With CEA or CAAS

We included three RCTs described in 11 publications[31,32,67-75] that compared CEA with medical therapy and 41 additional multi-institutional trials or cohort studies (including registries) that reported rates of relevant harms for either CEA or CAAS, regardless of the comparator. Of these, we rated 17 as poor quality, usually for high risk for selection bias and/or ascertainment bias. Characteristics and results of studies rated as poor quality are not described in detail in the main report; they are available in Appendix E Tables 2 and 3. Most studies reported perioperative death or stroke and did not report on other harms (e.g., nerve injuries, other postoperative harms, psychological harms).

Trial Characteristics

The RCTs comparing CEA with medical therapy are described in Table 2 and KQ 5. Characteristics of other included trials are presented in Table 4; these included four RCTs,[82-86] three uncontrolled trials,[87-89] one pooled analysis of two uncontrolled trials,[90] and one nonrandomized trial rated as poor quality.[91-93]

Two RCTs comparing CEA with different control groups that were not included in KQ 5 provide relevant rates of harms following CEA. The first, CASANOVA (Carotid Artery Stenosis with Asymptomatic Narrowing: Operation Versus Aspirin trial), was a multicenter RCT conducted in Germany in 410 patients randomized to CEA or control.[82] Nearly half of the patients randomized to the control group eventually received surgery due to development of 90 percent or greater stenosis in one artery, development of bilateral stenosis at 50 percent or greater, or development of symptomatic CAS.[82] The second trial, MACE (Mayo Asymptomatic Carotid Endarterectomy trial), compared low-dose aspirin with CEA and no aspirin.[83] MACE was terminated early because of high rates of MI and transient ischemic attack in the surgical group attributed to aspirin being withheld. We only included these two trials for the perioperative harms for the groups assigned to CEA. Both MACE and CASANOVA were conducted in the early 1990s in patients with 50 percent to 99 percent CAS, confirmed by angiography. Subjects in both trials were predominately male (56% to 63%) and most had hypertension (60% to 64%); 42 to 44 percent had CAD.

Two other multicenter RCTs compared CEA with CAAS: CREST (Carotid Revascularization Endarterectomy Versus Stenting Trial)[84,85] and SAPPHIRE (Stenting and Angioplasty with Protection in Patients at High Risk for Endarterectomy trial).[86] SAPPHIRE required that participants have at least one condition suggesting high surgical risk (e.g. age greater than 80 years, severe pulmonary disease, contralateral carotid occlusion). Participants were similar in the prevalence of hypertension (85% to 88%) and diabetes (25 to 33%). More subjects in SAPPHIRE had CAD than in CREST (81% vs. 44%). In both trials, interventionalists had to demonstrate low complication rates prior to participating.

Three studies used post-marketing surveillance data to provide rates following CAAS: two uncontrolled trials (CAPTURE [Carotid ACCULINK/ACCUNET Post Approval Trial to Uncover Rare Events trial] and CAPTURE-2)[87-89] and one pooled analysis of two uncontrolled trials (using CAPTURE-2 and EXACT [Emboshield® and Xact® Post Approval Carotid Stent Trial]).[90] The CAPTURE registry collected data prospectively from multiple sites that enrolled patients deemed high risk for surgery and who elected to undergo CAAS for asymptomatic stenosis.[87] Similarly, the CAPTURE-2 registry was a postapproval trial designed to capture rare events associated with CAAS.[88,89] All three studies had pre- and postintervention neurologic evaluation and independent adjudication of neurological outcomes. Across all three trials, the mean age of participants was 73 years, approximately 38 percent were female, a third had diabetes, approximately 90 percent had hypertension, and the mean degree of stenosis was 85 to 86 percent.

Observational Study Characteristics

Eight fair-quality, multi-institution cohort studies described in 12 publications reported perioperative harms of CEA (Table 4).[24,94-104] All eight used Medicare claims or enrollment databases to identify included populations; harms were identified using both claims data and medical chart review. Most were conducted in Medicare beneficiaries of single states,[24,96-104] and two studies used data from 10 states.[94,95]

One cohort conducted during the lead-in (credentialing) phase of CREST included rates of postoperative harms following CAAS cases prospectively submitted by 427 potential interventionalists prior to selecting operators for the CAAS arm of CREST.[105] The study reported data on 1,151 patients undergoing CAAS for asymptomatic CAS at 70 percent or greater, determined by angiography.

An additional eight fair-quality studies reported in-hospital (but not 30-day) perioperative events following CEA or CAAS (Table 4). Three utilized state discharge databases,[106-108] and five used the Nationwide Inpatient Sample (NIS).[109-113] The NIS data originates from a national survey of 20 percent of all nonfederal hospitals.[109,110] The results of these studies are provided in Table 5, with the results of the other studies rated as good or fair quality that reported rates of periprocedural harms, but are not included in this text because they only capture in-hospital events.

Sixteen other observational studies were rated as poor quality, usually due to high risk for selection bias and/or ascertainment bias. These included published data from the National Surgery Quality Improvement Program (NSQIP) database,[114-117] the Veteran's Administration NSQIP,[118,119] the Carotid Artery Revascularization and Endarterectomy (CARE) registry,[120,121] international registries,[122-126] and the Society for Vascular Surgery Vascular Registry (SVS-VR).[127-129] Additional details about the results and quality ratings of these studies are provided in Appendix D and E, respectively.

Trial Results

CEA compared with medical therapy. Table 3 summarizes the main results of the VACS, ACAS, and ACST. Appendix F includes complete results of our meta-analyses.

Perioperative (30-day) stroke or death. Our meta-analysis found that 1.9 percent more persons treated with CEA had perioperative stroke or death within 30 days compared with subjects in medical therapy groups (RD, 0.019 [95% CI, 0.012 to 0.026]).

Perioperative (30-day) nonfatal MI. Two of the trials reported this outcome. The ACST found a significant increase in events in subjects who were treated with CEA (10 events) compared with subjects who were treated with medical therapy (one event) (RD, 0.006 [95% CI, 0.002 to 0.010]). The VACS reported four events in the CEA group and none in the medical therapy group.

Age, sex, race, or ethnicity. None of the trials reported subgroup information by race or ethnicity. The ACAS and ACST provided some subgroup information for perioperative stroke or death. In ACAS, the crude rate of perioperative stroke or death was higher in women than men, but the difference was not statistically significant (3.6% vs. 1.7%, p=0.12). In ACST, the perioperative hazards of CEA did not differ by subgroups of age, sex, or extent of stenosis (data not reported).

Rates of perioperative harms after CEA or CAAS. Table 5 summarizes the main results of studies rated as good or fair quality that reported rates of periprocedural harms.

Perioperative (30-day) death or stroke after CEA. Our meta-analysis of seven cohort studies (n=17,474) that all used Medicare claims data and medical records found a rate of 3.3 percent (95% CI, 2.7 to 3.9) for death or stroke in the 30 days after CEA. Sensitivity analysis, including poor-quality cohort studies (including vascular registries and NSQIP data), found a rate of 2.8 percent; statistical heterogeneity was considerable (95% CI, 2.1 to 3.5; I^2 = 92.5%). This considerable heterogeneity was expected given the significant differences in sample selection, ascertainment methods, and quality.

In all trials that included a CEA arm, regardless of the comparator, the rate of 30-day death or stroke was 2.4 percent (95% CI, 1.7 to 3.1).

Perioperative (30-day) death or stroke after CAAS. One cohort study, the CREST lead-in, found a rate of 3.8 percent (95% CI, 2.86 to 5.09) for death or stroke in the 30 days after CAAS. Our meta-analysis of trials (n=6,152; 2 trials) found a rate of 3.1 percent (95% CI, 2.68 to 3.56).

Perioperative (30-day) MI after CEA. One cohort study including 1,378 Medicare beneficiaries undergoing CEA for asymptomatic CAS at six hospitals in New York state during 1997 to 1998 reported a 0.85 percent rate of nonfatal MI.[99] A similar study in Georgia Medicare beneficiaries (n=1,002) during 1993 reported a 0.8 percent rate of MI, and a 0.6 percent rate of MI-related death.[103] One RCT (CREST) reported a 2.2 percent rate of any MI following CEA.[85]

Perioperative (30-day) MI after CAAS. One RCT (CREST) reported a 1.2 percent rate of any MI in the 30 days following CAAS.[85]

Nerve injuries, infection, and other postoperative harms. In VACS, 3.8 percent of persons undergoing CEA (8 of 211) had cranial nerve injuries. Functional recovery was observed in all patients, and there was no permanent disability. The CASANOVA trial reported a 1.4 percent rate of lung embolism, 4.2 percent rate of permanent cranial nerve damage, 1.4 percent rate of pneumonia, and 2.8 percent rate of local hematoma requiring surgery in the 206 patients randomized to the immediate surgical arm.[82] The total frequency of major complications (e.g., death, stroke, minor stroke, MI, permanent cranial nerve damage) in the group randomized to immediate surgery was 7.9 percent. The MACE study reported a 1.1 percent rate of minor cranial nerve injury in the 36 patients randomized to CEA.[83]

Age, sex, race, or ethnicity. One cohort study (CREST lead-in) reported a 2.4 percent rate of perioperative death or stroke following CAAS for patients younger than age 75 years and 7.5 percent for persons older than age 75 years. It also reported a perioperative death, stroke, and MI rate of 3.3 percent for persons younger than age 75 years and 9.1 percent for persons older than age 75 years.[105]

In a pooled analysis of data from two uncontrolled trials (CAPTURE-2 and EXACT) the rate of death or stroke following CAAS in patients younger than age 80 years was 2.9 percent compared with a rate of 4.4 percent in persons age 80 years and older.[90]

Comorbidities. We found one fair-quality cohort study reporting rates of harms by comorbidity following CEA for asymptomatic CAS in 1998 and 1999. It reported a 30-day death or stroke rate of 7.13 percent in persons with high comorbidity versus 2.69 percent in persons with low comorbidity in Medicare beneficiaries at 150 hospitals in New York (6,932 patients).[24] High comorbidity was defined as any end-stage disease, severe disability, or three or more Revised Cardiac Risk Index risk factors (history of ischemic heart disease, congestive heart failure, stroke/transient ischemic attack, diabetes requiring insulin, creatinine >2, or undergoing a high-risk surgery).

Variation in rates of perioperative stroke or death following CEA by center volume. One study of Medicare beneficiaries who underwent CEA (350 procedures) during 1993 to 1994 in Oklahoma found a combined stroke and death rate at high-volume hospitals (>100 Medicare CEAs over the study period) of 3.5 percent, and a stroke and death rate at low-volume centers of 5.2 percent.[96]

A similar study of Medicare beneficiaries undergoing CEA at 115 hospitals in Ohio (167 procedures) reported a stroke or death rate of 0 percent at high-volume centers and 4.9 percent at low-volume centers during 1993 to 1994.[97]

Variation in rates of perioperative stroke or death following CEA by state. Two studies using cohorts of Medicare beneficiaries reported varying rates across 10 states.[94,95] Rates ranged from 2.3 to 6.7 percent using data from 1995 to 1996[95] and from 1.4 to 6.0 percent using data from 1998 to 1999.[94]

Chapter 4. Discussion

Summary of Evidence

No studies directly addressed our overarching question (KQ 1), and no studies randomly assigned patients, practices, or providers to screening and comparator groups and subsequently provided interventions for persons with positive screening results.

Detection of Asymptomatic CAS

Duplex ultrasonography is a widely available, noninvasive screening test with estimated sensitivity and specificity of 94 percent and 92 percent, respectively, for detecting CAS at 60 to 99 percent. Reliability of ultrasound is questionable, as accuracy can vary considerably between laboratories.

Use of duplex ultrasonography in a low-prevalence population would result in many false-positive tests. For example, in a population of 100,000 adults with an asymptomatic CAS prevalence of 1 percent, duplex ultrasonography would result in 940 true positives and 7,920 false positives (Table 6).

If no confirmatory tests are done and all persons with positive tests are referred for intervention, many unnecessary interventions and harms would occur. If all positive tests are followed by angiography (which is not typically done in clinical practice), up to 1.2 percent of persons will have a resulting stroke.[31] If all positive tests are followed by MRA (95% sensitivity and 90% specificity[47]), many patients would still be sent for unnecessary intervention. In the example above, 792 false positives would still be sent for intervention, almost as many as true positives sent for intervention (893).

If externally validated, reliable risk stratification tools were available to distinguish persons who are more likely to have CAS, allowing identification of a subset of the population with higher prevalence, then the ratio of true positives to false positives for screening with duplex ultrasonography (with or without confirmatory testing) would improve. However, the only study attempting external validation of such a tool found inadequate discrimination; it was little better than chance (c-statistic for ≥50% CAS, 0.60 [95% CI, 0.56 to 0.64]).

Benefits and Harms of Interventions for Asymptomatic CAS

An accurate estimate of overall benefit for the current general primary care population is difficult to obtain. Although our meta-analyses of RCTs comparing CEA with medical therapy found an absolute risk reduction of 3.5 percent for the composite of perioperative stroke or death or any subsequent stroke over approximately 5 years, the applicability of the evidence to current clinical practice is substantially limited. Medical therapy was often not clearly defined or standardized, was not kept constant during the study, and would not have included treatments now considered to be current standard medical therapy, including aggressive management of blood pressure and lipids. To address some applicability limitations of previous studies, including those related to current standard medical therapy, the new CREST-2 trial[130] (enrollment to begin in 2014) will compare both a) CAAS with medical therapy versus medical therapy alone and b) CEA with medical therapy versus medical therapy alone. None of the identified trials focused on a population found by screening in primary care. Definitions of asymptomatic status varied across the trials and included subjects with a history of contralateral stroke or transient ischemic attack (25% in ACAS; 32% in VACS; not reported in ACST), nonrecent ipsilateral symptoms, and prior contralateral CEA.

The trials comparing CEA with medical therapy used highly selected surgeons, requiring low rates of complications to allow participation, and stipulated no further enrollment by surgeons or institutions that showed unacceptably high morbidity or mortality during the trial, providing some disincentive to report harms. A relatively low perioperative stroke or death rate is required for CEA to have a reasonable likelihood of resulting in more benefit than harm for persons with asymptomatic CAS; overall benefit depends on surviving the perioperative period without experiencing significant harms. Our meta-analyses of trial data found 30-day perioperative rates of stroke or death of 2.4 percent for CEA and 3.1 percent for CAAS. Observational data suggest higher rates: 3.3 percent for CEA and 3.8 percent for CAAS. Observational data also revealed a wide range of these rates for CEA across states, as high as 6.7 percent in some states.[95]

The potential benefits of CEA or CAAS depend on the risk for an asymptomatic lesion eventually resulting in a stroke, and evidence from systematic reviews suggests that this risk has decreased in recent decades, most likely due to advances in medical therapy.[78,131] The best recent evidence suggests that the incidence rate of ipsilateral stroke is nearing 1 percent per year,[78] approaching the rate achieved in the surgical arms of trials comparing CEA with medical therapy. This would significantly reduce the potential benefits of surgery. Current medical intervention alone has also been estimated to be three to eight times more cost effective.[131]

In theory, patients at higher risk for ipsilateral stroke might be more likely to benefit from surgery or intervention. However, no externally validated, reliable risk stratification tools are available that can distinguish persons with asymptomatic CAS who are at decreased or increased risk for stroke caused by CAS, despite current standard medical therapy, or for persons at decreased or increased risk for harms from CEA or CAAS. One might expect that persons with greater reduction of the carotid diameter would have greater potential for benefit (e.g., perhaps persons with 80% to 99% CAS vs. 60% to 79% CAS), but subgroup analyses from trials comparing CEA with medical therapy found no significant difference by percent CAS.[31,32]

Notably, the main estimates of overall benefit (i.e., perioperative stroke or death or any subsequent stroke) from the trials comparing CEA with medical therapy do not include some important harms, such as nonfatal MI. More recently published head-to-head trials comparing CEA and CAAS used composite primary outcomes that include periprocedural MI.[84,86] The trials comparing CEA with medical therapy reported rates of perioperative nonfatal MI of 0.7 percent (ACST) to 1.9 percent (VACS).

Other important harms reported in trials or observational studies include permanent cranial nerve damage, pulmonary embolism, pneumonia, wound infection, acute renal failure, urinary tract infection, deep venous thrombosis, and local hematoma requiring surgery. Most studies we reviewed did not report on harms other than perioperative stroke or death. Thus, lack of reporting or underreporting of some harms is possible. Some studies with more detailed reporting of harms suggest higher rates of major complications from surgery compared with ACAS, ACST, and VACS. For example, 7.9 percent of participants randomized to CEA in the CASANOVA trial reported at least one major complication (including death, stroke, pulmonary embolism, MI, or permanent cranial nerve damage). It is unclear whether these seemingly high rates were identified due to a more complete ascertainment of harms or for other reasons. Studies using NSQIP data from 2005 to 2007 reported rates for peripheral nerve injury (0.32%), wound infection (0.68%), pneumonia (0.66%),[114] and for wound disruption, unplanned intubation, pulmonary embolism, acute renal failure, urinary tract infection, deep venous thrombosis, and sepsis (<1% each).[115] Although we rated the studies using NSQIP data as poor quality, primarily due to high risk for selection bias and ascertainment bias, we were concerned that rates of some harms reported in these studies underestimate, rather than overestimate, actual rates of harms.

Timing of events is another important concept not addressed by the main estimates of overall benefit reported in trials of CEA compared with medical therapy. Consolidating all stroke and death events together into one composite outcome does not reflect different values that patients may have for a stroke or death caused by surgery than for a stroke or death that is caused by natural progression.

Life expectancy is another important consideration when assessing the potential for overall benefit. Based on the data from randomized trials, a life expectancy of at least 5 years would be needed to have a reasonable chance of benefit of CEA. Somewhat related are issues associated with advanced age (older than 75 years). Potential for benefit decreases with advanced age because of competing hazards. The mean age of patients in trials comparing CEA with medical therapy was in the mid- to upper-60s. But, the mean age of Medicare patients undergoing CEA is 75 years,[23] raising the question of whether many persons having surgical intervention are likely too old to benefit.

Potential Psychological Harms of Screening for CAS

The CAS screening cascade has potential psychological harms. Anxiety and distress occur frequently after positive screening tests for many conditions;[132-134] this result may also occur after positive ultrasound screening for CAS. At least some of these positive screening tests will be false positives. The longer-term experience of persons with false-positive results is unknown. Some persons may have a "near positive" Doppler screening test. In these situations, standard clinical practice will likely involve surveillance over time, with repeated ultrasound testing to determine a point where intervention might be considered. The psychological effect of this surveillance—prolonging the period of uncertainty before resolution—is potentially problematic, although unstudied.

In addition to false-positive screening tests, some persons who would have never had a cerebrovascular event will receive positive confirmatory tests and/or proceed to CEA or CAAS. These persons will have been overdiagnosed and, likely, overtreated[135,136] with CEA or CAAS to prevent a problem from which they never would have suffered. In addition to the obvious potential physical harms involved, important psychological harms are possible. Diagnosing a person with CAS may lead to anxiety about the possibility of having a stroke; it may also lead to intrusive thoughts and distraction about the future, thus disturbing quality of life. If prevalence of CAS is about 1 percent, then many more persons will likely experience overdiagnosis than will avoid a stroke. We were unable to find research describing the frequency of these important potential psychological harms.

Hypothetical Outcomes of a General Population Screening Program

The hypothetical outcomes of a screening program for asymptomatic CAS in the general population are illustrated in Table 6. Assumptions used to determine the hypothetical outcomes include a CAS prevalence of 1 percent and the use of duplex ultrasonography as the screening test followed by confirmatory testing with MRA; this strategy results in a better ratio of benefits to harms than no confirmatory testing or angiography confirmation (i.e., best possible scenario for screening to show overall benefit[2]). A detailed list of assumptions is provided below Table 6. Hypothetical outcomes were calculated using both trial and cohort results. Trial data for benefits and harms suggest that nine major cardiovascular events (composite of perioperative stroke, death, MI, and any subsequent stroke) would be prevented over 5 years by screening 100,000 persons and intervening with CEA. Trial data estimates for benefits and observational data for estimates of harms found that screening followed by CEA resulted in net harm (19 more events). The hypothetical outcomes likely overestimate the potential benefits of CEA because the estimates of benefit come from trials that did not compare CEA with current standard medical therapy. Further, the number needed to screen and the net for major cardiovascular events do not include cranial nerve injuries, other complications of surgery (pulmonary embolism, pneumonia, other infection, local hematoma requiring surgery), or potential psychological harms.

Auscultation for Carotid Bruit

In 1996, the USPSTF concluded that auscultation for carotid bruits has low sensitivity and specificity and considerable interobserver variation in the interpretation of key auditory characteristics.[137] Assessment of carotid bruits was not included in the 2007 systematic review because it was determined that the evidence had likely not changed appreciably.[1,2] We searched the literature covering 1996 to early 2013 and found no evidence that auscultation has improved as a screening tool to detect clinically significant levels of asymptomatic CAS. We identified four studies reporting screening accuracy by auscultation.[138-141] Minimum cutoff values for CAS ranged from 50 to 70 percent. All studies used ultrasound as the gold standard for comparison; none used angiography. The reported sensitivities ranged from 46 to 77 percent, and specificities ranged from 71 to 98 percent. Only two studies involved patients from the general population (one in the United States[138] and the other in France);[139] one study included Swedish patients referred to a hospital for carotid surgery investigation,[140] and the fourth study was in Chinese patients with peripheral vascular disease.[141]

Limitations

The limitations primarily reflect the published literature. We found no eligible studies addressing our overarching question (KQ 1), questions about externally validated, reliable risk stratification tools to distinguish persons with asymptomatic CAS who have increased or decreased risk for ipsilateral stroke or of harms after CEA or CAAS (KQ 4), and whether additional medications (e.g., aspirin, statins) provide incremental benefit beyond current standard medical therapy including treatment of traditional risk factors (e.g., hypertension, hypercholesterolemia)—that is, we found no evidence that the potential to intensify medical therapy justifies screening for CAS (KQ 6).

Most key issues limiting the applicability of the evidence are described in the Discussion above: no trials compared CEA or CAAS with current standard medical therapy, trials used highly selected surgeons and participants, certain perioperative harms may be underreported, and applicability of the trial evidence to the general asymptomatic primary care population is limited.

Most evidence focused on CEA. We found no trials comparing CAAS with medical therapy. Head-to-head trials have reported that CAAS was not inferior to CEA in high-risk patients for a composite outcome (death, stroke, or MI within 30 days of intervention or death or ipsilateral stroke between 31 days and 1 year; SAPPHIRE, n=334)[86] or that the two interventions did not differ significantly for a slightly different composite outcome (stroke, MI, or death from any cause during the periprocedural period or any ipsilateral stroke within 4 years; CREST, n=2,502).[84] Several critics have explained why CREST does not actually demonstrate equivalence of CEA and CAAS and why it actually shows that CAAS is more risky than CEA.[142,143] For example, mostly minor MIs (that occurred more frequently in the CAS group) were given equal weight to strokes and death in the periprocedural composite endpoint, but not in the 4-year, long-term endpoint (and the CAAS group had more MIs over the long-term).[142]

Some changes in technology, standard medical therapy, surgical procedures, and stroke rates may not be reflected in some of the included literature (e.g., studies conducted in the 1990s). Recent reviews and meta-analyses found moderate strength of evidence that standard medical therapy has reduced the rate of ipsilateral stroke over time.[131,143,144] Our review did not evaluate the use of carotid intima-media thickness in assessing coronary heart disease risk, but a previous review for the USPSTF concluded that evidence does not support its use.[145]

The single study we identified for KQ 2 had several important limitations. The study tested relatively basic prediction tools: simple and weighted scores. Multivariate modeling is likely to produce more robust prediction. Next, the scores used a limited number of predictive variables. Testing inclusion of additional and alternate clinical variables will be important to improve predictive ability. Finally, it used a limited set of validation measures. Testing calibration (the ability of the tool to correctly categorize risk compared with observed events) as well as discrimination (the ability of the tool to correctly classify persons with disease at higher risk than persons without disease) would provide a better sense of the model's utility in clinical practice.

Future Research Needs

Good-quality studies are needed to establish: 1) an externally validated, reliable risk stratification tool to identify populations with higher prevalence of CAS; 2) improved screening strategies for CAS that generate fewer false-positive results and unnecessary harms; 3) an externally validated, reliable risk stratification tool to distinguish persons who are more likely to benefit after intervention from persons who are more likely to be harmed; and 4) the comparative benefits and harms of current standard medical therapy, CEA, and CAAS.

Even if future research develops externally validated, reliable risk stratification tools that identify populations with higher prevalence of CAS, such tools would not be sufficient to warrant routine screening for asymptomatic CAS. Given the limitations of the applicability of ACST, ACAS, and VACS, new trials would be needed to establish whether surgery or intervention have overall benefit over current standard medical therapy for the higher prevalence population.[131] Similar limitations apply to risk stratification tools that distinguish persons who are more likely to benefit after intervention from persons who are more likely to be harmed.

Although we found no externally validated, reliable risk stratification tools addressing KQ 4, we identified publications that derive risk prediction tools that could be informative for future research or could be targets for future external validation.[60-66] These tools included risk factors and are focused on various outcomes. We did not critically appraise these publications, and they may have important limitations. We also identified risk factor studies, particularly for associations between clinical or radiologic factors and stroke outcomes in persons with known CAS. These studies suggest multiple variables beyond the traditional risk factors that should be considered for inclusion and testing in risk prediction models developed in the future (e.g., plaque characteristics, genetic markers, embolic signal detection[146-150]). Future studies should use a variety of validation measures.

Our searches of clinical trial registries identified four trials that are ongoing or not yet published comparing CEA or CAAS with medical therapy (AMTEC [Aggressive Medical Treatment Evaluation for Asymptomatic Carotid Artery Stenosis, NCT00805311], SPACE-2 [Stent-Protected Angioplasty in Asymptomatic Carotid Artery Stenosis vs. Endarterectomy: Two Two-Arm Clinical Trials, ISRCTN78592017], ECST-2 [ISRCTN97744893], and NCT00497094) and three comparing CEA with CAAS (ACT-1 [Carotid Stenting vs. Surgery of Severe Carotid Artery Disease and Stroke Prevention in Asymptomatic Patients, NCT00106938], ACST-2 [NCT00883402], and NCT00772278).

Despite the potential future research we suggested above, these needs may be relatively low priority considering that the potential preventable burden of disease is fairly low from a larger resource and public health perspective. Several studies have illustrated that patients with asymptomatic CAS are more likely to suffer MI or nonstroke vascular deaths than ipsilateral stroke, suggesting that preventive strategies for these patients should perhaps concentrate on coronary risk more than stroke.[20] In ACST, about five times as many nonstroke vascular deaths as nonperioperative stroke deaths were observed (267 and 68 deaths for the medical therapy group, respectively; 298 and 39 for the CEA group, respectively).[32]

Response to Public Comment

A draft version of this report was posted for public comment on the USPSTF Web site from February 18 to March 17, 2014. We received a comment from one clinician. The commenter thought that the report should consider that the ability of carotid ultrasound to detect the atherosclerotic process could lead to earlier initiation or intensification of medical therapy and ultimately to better outcomes. We attempted to evaluate evidence of such possible benefit with KQ 6, but we found no evidence that the potential to intensify medical therapy justifies screening for CAS. Thus, we did not make changes to the report in response to the comment.

The commenter also recommended that there should be a caveat for patients at higher risk. However, externally validated, reliable risk stratification tools are not available.

Conclusion

Asymptomatic CAS has low prevalence in the general adult population. Noninvasive screening with ultrasound would result in many false-positive results; confirmatory testing with MRA appears to be the best strategy to optimize benefits and harms (compared with no confirmatory testing or angiography confirmation), but still yields a significant number of false-positive results. Externally validated, reliable risk stratification tools to distinguish persons who are more likely to have CAS are not available. Furthermore, current evidence does not sufficiently establish incremental overall benefit of CEA beyond current standard medical therapy, primarily because medical therapy in trials was ill-defined, varying, and often lacked treatments that are now standard. Advances in medical therapy have reduced the rate of stroke in persons with asymptomatic CAS in recent decades. No RCTs compared CAAS with medical therapy. Externally validated, reliable risk stratification tools that can distinguish persons with asymptomatic CAS who have increased or decreased risk for ipsilateral stroke or harms after CEA or CAAS are not available.

References

1.   Wolff T, Guirguis-Blake J, Miller T, et al. Screening for Asymptomatic Carotid Artery Stenosis. Evidence Synthesis No. 50. AHRQ Publication No. 08-05102-EF-1. Rockville, MD: Agency for Healthcare Research and Quality; 2007.

2.   Wolff T, Guirguis-Blake J, Miller T, et al. Screening for carotid artery stenosis: an update of the evidence for the U.S. Preventive Services Task Force. *Ann Intern Med.* 2007;147(12):860-70. PMID: 18087057.

3.   U.S. Preventive Services Task Force. Screening for carotid artery stenosis: U.S. Preventive Services Task Force recommendation statement. *Ann Intern Med.* 2007;147(12):854-9. PMID: 18087056.

4.   Hall H. Ultrasound screening: misleading the public. 2008 http://www.sciencebasedmedicine.org/ultrasound-screening-misleading-the-public. Accessed on October 18, 2013.

5.   Kochanek KD, Xu J, Murphy SL, et al. Deaths: Final Data for 2009.. Hyattsville, MD: National Center for Health Statistics; 2011. http://www.cdc.gov/nchs/data/nvsr60/nvsr60_03.pdf.

6.   Roger VL, Go AS, Lloyd-Jones DM, et al. Heart disease and stroke statistics—2012 update: a report from the American Heart Association. *Circulation.* 2012;125(1):e2-e220. PMID: 22179539.

7.   Centers for Disease Control and Prevention. Prevalence of stroke—United States, 2006-2010. *MMWR Morb Mortal Wkly Rep.* 2012;61(20):379-82. PMID: 22622094.

8.   Kistler JP, Furie KL. Carotid endarterectomy revisited. *N Engl J Med.* 2000;342(23):1743-5. PMID: 10841879.

9.   Centers for Disease Control and Prevention. Prevalence and most common causes of disability among adults—United States, 2005. *MMWR Morb Mortal Wkly Rep.* 2009;58(16):421-6. PMID: 19407734.

10.   Kelly-Hayes M, Beiser A, Kase CS, et al. The influence of gender and age on disability following ischemic stroke: the Framingham study. *J Stroke Cerebrovasc Dis.* 2003;12(3):119-26. PMID: 17903915.

11.   Brown DL, Boden-Albala B, Langa KM, et al. Projected costs of ischemic stroke in the United States. *Neurology.* 2006;67(8):1390-5. PMID: 16914694.

12.   de Weerd M, Greving JP, de Jong AW, et al. Prevalence of asymptomatic carotid artery stenosis according to age and sex: systematic review and metaregression analysis. *Stroke.* 2009;40(4):1105-13. PMID: 19246704.

13.   O'Leary DH, Polak JF, Kronmal RA, et al. Distribution and correlates of sonographically detected carotid artery disease in the Cardiovascular Health Study. The CHS Collaborative Research Group. *Stroke.* 1992;23(12):1752-60. PMID: 1448826.

14.   Longstreth WT, Jr., Shemanski L, Lefkowitz D, et al. Asymptomatic internal carotid artery stenosis defined by ultrasound and the risk of subsequent stroke in the elderly. The Cardiovascular Health Study. *Stroke.* 1998;29(11):2371-6. PMID: 9804651.

15.   Lewis RF, Abrahamowicz M, Cote R, et al. Predictive power of duplex ultrasonography in asymptomatic carotid disease. *Ann Intern Med.* 1997;127(1):13-20. PMID: 9214247.

16. Muluk SC, Muluk VS, Sugimoto H, et al. Progression of asymptomatic carotid stenosis: a natural history study in 1004 patients. *J Vasc Surg*. 1999;29(2):208-14; discussion 14-6. PMID: 9950979.

17. Mansour MA, Mattos MA, Faught WE, et al. The natural history of moderate (50% to 79%) internal carotid artery stenosis in symptomatic, nonhemispheric, and asymptomatic patients. *J Vasc Surg*. 1995;21(2):346-56; discussion 56-7. PMID: 7853606.

18. Nehler MR, Moneta GL, Lee RW, et al. Improving selection of patients with less than 60% asymptomatic internal carotid artery stenosis for follow-up carotid artery duplex scanning. *J Vasc Surg*. 1996;24(4):580-5; discussion 5-7. PMID: 8911406.

19. Rockman CB, Riles TS, Lamparello PJ, et al. Natural history and management of the asymptomatic, moderately stenotic internal carotid artery. *J Vasc Surg*. 1997;25(3):423-31. PMID: 9081121.

20. Nadareishvili ZG, Rothwell PM, Beletsky V, et al. Long-term risk of stroke and other vascular events in patients with asymptomatic carotid artery stenosis. *Arch Neurol*. 2002;59(7):1162-6. PMID: 12117365.

21. Goldstein LB, Bushnell CD, Adams RJ, et al. Guidelines for the primary prevention of stroke: a guideline for healthcare professionals from the American Heart Association/American Stroke Association. *Stroke*. 2011;42(2):517-84. PMID: 21127304.

22. Makris GC, Lavida A, Nicolaides AN, et al. The effect of statins on carotid plaque morphology: a LDL-associated action or one more pleiotropic effect of statins? *Atherosclerosis*. 2010;213(1):8-20. PMID: 20494361.

23. Patel MR, Greiner MA, DiMartino LD, et al. Geographic variation in carotid revascularization among Medicare beneficiaries, 2003-2006. *Arch Intern Med*. 2010;170(14):1218-25. PMID: 20660840.

24. Halm EA, Tuhrim S, Wang JJ, et al. Has evidence changed practice?: appropriateness of carotid endarterectomy after the clinical trials. *Neurology*. 2007;68(3):187-94. PMID: 17224571.

25. Kansara A, Miller D, Damani R, et al. Variability in carotid endarterectomy practice patterns within a metropolitan area. *Stroke*. 2012;43(11):3105-7. PMID: 22933589.

26. Nallamothu BK, Lu M, Rogers MA, et al. Physician specialty and carotid stenting among elderly medicare beneficiaries in the United States. *Arch Intern Med*. 2011;171(20):1804-10. PMID: 21824938.

27. Methods Guide for Effectiveness and Comparative Effectiveness Reviews. AHRQ Publication No. 10(11)-EHC063-EF. Rockville: MD: Agency for Healthcare Research and Quality; 2011. Chapters available at: http://www.effectivehealthcare.ahrq.gov.

28. Harris RP, Helfand M, Woolf SH, et al. Current methods of the US Preventive Services Task Force: a review of the process. *Am J Prev Med*. 2001;20(3 Suppl):21-35. PMID: 11306229.

29. West SL, Gartlehner G, Mansfield AJ, et al. Comparative Effectiveness Review Methods: Clinical Heterogeneity. Methods Research Report. AHRQ Publication No. 10-EHC070-EF. Rockville, MD: Agency for Healthcare Research and Quality; 2010.

30. Sutton AJ, Abrams KR, Jones DR, et al. Methods for Meta-Analysis in Medical Research (Wiley Series in Probability and Statistics - Applied Probability and Statistics Section). London: Wiley; 2000.

31. Endarterectomy for asymptomatic carotid artery stenosis. Executive Committee for the Asymptomatic Carotid Atherosclerosis Study. *JAMA*. 1995;273(18):1421-8. PMID: 7723155.

32. Halliday A, Harrison M, Hayter E, et al. 10-year stroke prevention after successful carotid endarterectomy for asymptomatic stenosis (ACST-1): a multicentre randomised trial. *Lancet*. 2010;376(9746):1074-84. PMID: 20870099.

33. Wilson EB. Probable inference, the law of succession, and statistical inference. *J Am Stat Assoc*. 1927;22:209-12.

34. Higgins JP, Thompson SG. Quantifying heterogeneity in a meta-analysis. *Stat Med*. 2002;21(11):1539-58. PMID: 12111919.

35. Higgins JP, Thompson SG, Deeks JJ, et al. Measuring inconsistency in meta-analyses. *BMJ*. 2003;327(7414):557-60. PMID: 12958120.

36. Higgins JPT, Green ST, eds. Cochrane Handbook for Systematic Reviews of Interventions Version 5.1.0: The Cochrane Collaboration. Available from www.cochrane-handbook.org; Updated March 2011.

37. Kontopantelis E, Reeves D. metaan: Random-effects meta-analysis. *Stata J*. 2010;10(3):395-407.

38. Kontopantelis E, Springate DA, Reeves D. A re-analysis of the Cochrane Library data: the dangers of unobserved heterogeneity in meta-analyses. *PLoS One*. 2013;8(7):e69930. PMID: 23922860.

39. Hardy RJ, Thompson SG. A likelihood approach to meta-analysis with random effects. *Stat Med*. 1996;15(6):619-29. PMID: 8731004.

40. Jackson D, White IR, Thompson SG. Extending DerSimonian and Laird's methodology to perform multivariate random effects meta-analyses. *Stat Med*. 2010;29(12):1282-97. PMID: 19408255.

41. Suri MF, Ezzeddine MA, Lakshminarayan K, et al. Validation of two different grading schemes to identify patients with asymptomatic carotid artery stenosis in general population. *J Neuroimaging*. 2008;18(2):142-7. PMID: 18380694.

42. Jacobowitz GR, Rockman CB, Gagne PJ, et al. A model for predicting occult carotid artery stenosis: screening is justified in a selected population. *J Vasc Surg*. 2003;38(4):705-9. PMID: 14560217.

43. Qureshi AI, Janardhan V, Bennett SE, et al. Who should be screened for asymptomatic carotid artery stenosis? Experience from the Western New York Stroke Screening Program. *J Neuroimaging*. 2001;11(2):105-11. PMID: 11296578.

44. Lloyd-Jones DM. Cardiovascular risk prediction: basic concepts, current status, and future directions. *Circulation*. 2010;121(15):1768-77. PMID: 20404268.

45. Hosmer DW, Lemeshow S. Applied Logistic Regression. New York, NY: John Wiley & Sons; 2000.

46. Jahromi AS, Cina CS, Liu Y, et al. Sensitivity and specificity of color duplex ultrasound measurement in the estimation of internal carotid artery stenosis: a systematic review and meta-analysis. *J Vasc Surg*. 2005;41(6):962-72. PMID: 15944595.

47. Nederkoorn PJ, Graaf Y, Hunink M. Duplex ultrasound and magnetic resonance angiography compared with digital subtraction angiography in carotid artery stenosis: a systematic review (structured abstract). *Stroke*. 2003;34(5):1324-31. PMID: DARE-12003000974.

48.   Blakeley DD, Oddone EZ, Hasselblad V, et al. Noninvasive carotid artery testing. A meta-analytic review. *Ann Intern Med*. 1995;122(5):360-7. PMID: 7847648.

49.   Jogestrand T, Lindqvist M, Nowak J. Diagnostic performance of duplex ultrasonography in the detection of high grade internal carotid artery stenosis. *Eur J Vasc Endovasc Surg*. 2002;23(6):510-8. PMID: 12093067.

50.   Nowak J, Jogestrand T. Duplex ultrasonography is an efficient diagnostic tool for the detection of moderate to severe internal carotid artery stenosis. *Clin Physiol Funct Imaging*. 2007;27(3):144-7. PMID: 17445064.

51.   Sabeti S, Schillinger M, Mlekusch W, et al. Quantification of internal carotid artery stenosis with duplex US: comparative analysis of different flow velocity criteria. *Radiology*. 2004;232(2):431-9. PMID: 15286315.

52.   Hwang CS, Liao KM, Lee JH, et al. Measurement of carotid stenosis: comparisons between duplex and different angiographic grading methods. *J Neuroimaging*. 2003;13(2):133-9. PMID: 12722495.

53.   Rothwell PM, Gibson RJ, Slattery J, et al. Equivalence of measurements of carotid stenosis. A comparison of three methods on 1001 angiograms. European Carotid Surgery Trialists' Collaborative Group. *Stroke*. 1994;25(12):2435-9. PMID: 7974586.

54.   Rothwell PM, Gutnikov SA, Warlow CP. Reanalysis of the final results of the European Carotid Surgery Trial. *Stroke*. 2003;34(2):514-23. PMID: 12574569.

55.   Hoskins PR. A review of the measurement of blood velocity and related quantities using Doppler ultrasound. *Proc Inst Mech Eng H*. 1999;213(5):391-400. PMID: 10581966.

56.   Nicolaides AN, Shifrin EG, Bradbury A, et al. Angiographic and duplex grading of internal carotid stenosis: can we overcome the confusion? *J Endovasc Surg*. 1996;3(2):158-65. PMID: 8798134.

57.   Tola M, Yurdakul M. Effect of Doppler angle in diagnosis of internal carotid artery stenosis. *J Ultrasound Med*. 2006;25(9):1187-92. PMID: 16929020.

58.   Kuntz KM, Polak JF, Whittemore AD, et al. Duplex ultrasound criteria for the identification of carotid stenosis should be laboratory specific. *Stroke*. 1997;28(3):597-602. PMID: 9056618.

59.   Alexandrov AV, Vital D, Brodie DS, et al. Grading carotid stenosis with ultrasound. An interlaboratory comparison. *Stroke*. 1997;28(6):1208-10. PMID: 9183353.

60.   Nicolaides AN, Kakkos SK, Kyriacou E, et al. Asymptomatic internal carotid artery stenosis and cerebrovascular risk stratification. *J Vasc Surg*. 2010;52(6):1486-96 e1-5. PMID: 21146746.

61.   Calvillo-King L, Xuan L, Zhang S, et al. Predicting risk of perioperative death and stroke after carotid endarterectomy in asymptomatic patients: derivation and validation of a clinical risk score. *Stroke*. 2010;41(12):2786-94. PMID: 21051669.

62.   Goodney PP, Likosky DS, Cronenwett JL. Factors associated with stroke or death after carotid endarterectomy in Northern New England. *J Vasc Surg*. 2008;48(5):1139-45. PMID: 18586446.

63.   Bertges DJ, Goodney PP, Zhao Y, et al. The Vascular Study Group of New England Cardiac Risk Index (VSG-CRI) predicts cardiac complications more accurately than the Revised Cardiac Risk Index in vascular surgery patients. *J Vasc Surg*. 2010;52(3):674-83, 83 e1-83 e3. PMID: 20570467.

64. Momjian-Mayor I, Kuzmanovic I, Momjian S, et al. Accuracy of a novel risk index combining degree of stenosis of the carotid artery and plaque surface echogenicity. *Stroke*. 2012;43(5):1260-5. PMID: 22403049.

65. Prati P, Tosetto A, Casaroli M, et al. Carotid plaque morphology improves stroke risk prediction: usefulness of a new ultrasonographic score. *Cerebrovasc Dis*. 2011;31(3):300-4. PMID: 21212660.

66. Folkersen L, Persson J, Ekstrand J, et al. Prediction of ischemic events on the basis of transcriptomic and genomic profiling in patients undergoing carotid endarterectomy. *Mol Med*. 2012;18:669-75. PMID: 22371308.

67. Halliday A, Mansfield A, Marro J, et al. Prevention of disabling and fatal strokes by successful carotid endarterectomy in patients without recent neurological symptoms: randomised controlled trial. *Lancet*. 2004;363(9420):1491-502. PMID: 15135594.

68. Halliday AW, Thomas D, Mansfield A. The Asymptomatic Carotid Surgery Trial (ACST). Rationale and design. Steering Committee. *Eur J Vasc Surg*. 1994;8(6):703-10. PMID: 7828747.

69. Halliday AW, Thomas DJ, Mansfield AO. The asymptomatic carotid surgery trial (ACST). *Int angiol*. 1995;14(1):18-20. PMID: 7658099.

70. Young B, Moore WS, Robertson JT, et al. An analysis of perioperative surgical mortality and morbidity in the asymptomatic carotid atherosclerosis study. *Stroke*. 1996;27(12):2216-24. PMID: 8969784.

71. Baker WH, Howard VJ, Howard G, et al. Effect of contralateral occlusion on long-term efficacy of endarterectomy in the asymptomatic carotid atherosclerosis study (ACAS). ACAS Investigators. *Stroke*. 2000;31(10):2330-4. PMID: 11022059.

72. Asymptomatic Carotid Atherosclerosis Study Group. Study design for randomized prospective trial of carotid endarterectomy for asymptomatic atherosclerosis. *Stroke*. 1989;20(7):844-9. PMID: 2665205.

73. Hobson RW, 2nd, Weiss DG, Fields WS, et al. Efficacy of carotid endarterectomy for asymptomatic carotid stenosis. The Veterans Affairs Cooperative Study Group. *N Engl J Med*. 1993;328(4):221-7. PMID: 8418401.

74. Towne JB, Weiss DG, Hobson RW. First phase report of cooperative Veterans Administration asymptomatic carotid stenosis study—operative morbidity and mortality. *J Vasc Surg*. 1990;11(2):252-8; discussion 8-9. PMID: 2405197.

75. Role of carotid endarterectomy in asymptomatic carotid stenosis. A Veterans Administration Cooperative Study. *Stroke*. 1986;17(3):534-9. PMID: 2872740.

76. den Hartog AG, Halliday AW, Hayter E, et al. Risk of stroke from new carotid artery occlusion in the Asymptomatic Carotid Surgery Trial-1. *Stroke*. 2013;44(6):1652-9. PMID: 23632980.

77. Chambers BR, Donnan GA. Carotid endarterectomy for asymptomatic carotid stenosis. *Cochrane Database Syst Rev*. 2005(4):CD001923. PMID: 16235289.

78. Raman G, Moorthy D, Hadar N, et al. Management strategies for asymptomatic carotid stenosis: a systematic review and meta-analysis. *Ann Intern Med*. 2013;158(9):676-85. PMID: 23648949.

79. Raman G, Kitsios GD, Moorthy D, et al. Management of Asymptomatic Carotid Artery Stenosis. Technology Assessment Report. Rockville, MD: Agency for Healthcare Research and Quality; 2012.

80. Benavente O, Moher D, Pham B. Carotid endarterectomy for asymptomatic carotid stenosis: a meta-analysis. *BMJ*. 1998;317(7171):1477-80. PMID: 9831572.

81. Guay J, Ochroch EA. Carotid endarterectomy plus medical therapy or medical therapy alone for carotid artery stenosis in symptomatic or asymptomatic patients: a meta-analysis (Structured abstract). *Cardiothorac Vasc Anesth*. 2012;26(5):835-44.

82. Carotid surgery versus medical therapy in asymptomatic carotid stenosis. The CASANOVA Study Group. Stroke. 1991;22(10):1229-35. PMID: 1926232.

83. Wiebers DO. Results of a randomized controlled trial of carotid endarterectomy for asymptomatic carotid stenosis. *Mayo Clin Proc*. 1992;67(6):513-8.

84. Brott TG, Hobson RW, 2nd, Howard G, et al. Stenting versus endarterectomy for treatment of carotid-artery stenosis. *N Engl J Med*. 2010;363(1):11-23. PMID: 20505173.

85. Silver FL, Mackey A, Clark WM, et al. Safety of stenting and endarterectomy by symptomatic status in the Carotid Revascularization Endarterectomy Versus Stenting Trial (CREST). *Stroke*. 2011;42(3):675-80. PMID: 21307169.

86. Yadav JS, Wholey MH, Kuntz RE, et al. Protected carotid-artery stenting versus endarterectomy in high-risk patients. *N Engl J Med*. 2004;351(15):1493-501. PMID: 15470212.

87. Fairman R, Gray WA, Scicli AP, et al. The CAPTURE registry: analysis of strokes resulting from carotid artery stenting in the post approval setting: timing, location, severity, and type. *Ann Surg*. 2007;246(4):551-6; discussion 6-8. PMID: 17893491.

88. Chaturvedi S, Matsumura JS, Gray W, et al. Carotid artery stenting in octogenarians: periprocedural stroke risk predictor analysis from the multicenter Carotid ACCULINK/ACCUNET Post Approval Trial to Uncover Rare Events (CAPTURE 2) clinical trial. *Stroke*. 2010;41(4):757-64. PMID: 20185789.

89. Matsumura JS, Gray W, Chaturvedi S, et al. CAPTURE 2 risk-adjusted stroke outcome benchmarks for carotid artery stenting with distal embolic protection. *J Vasc Surg*. 2010;52(3):576-83, 83 e1-83 e2. PMID: 20576398.

90. Gray WA, Chaturvedi S, Verta P. Thirty-day outcomes for carotid artery stenting in 6320 patients from 2 prospective, multicenter, high-surgical-risk registries. *Circ Cardiovasc Interv*. 2009;2(3):159-66. PMID: 20031712.

91. CaRESS Steering Committee. Carotid revascularization using endarterectomy or stenting systems (CARESS): Phase I clinical trial. *J Endovasc Ther*. 2003;10(6):1021-30. PMID: 14723574.

92. White RA, Diethrich E, Fogarty TJ, et al. Carotid Revascularization Using Endarterectomy or Stenting Systems (CaRESS) phase I clinical trial: 1-Year results. *J Vasc Surg*. 2005;42(2):213-9. PMID: 16102616.

93. Zarins CK, White RA, Diethrich EB, et al. Carotid revascularization using endarterectomy or stenting systems (CaRESS): 4-year outcomes. *J Endovasc Ther*. 2009;16(4):397-409. PMID: 19702339.

94. Kresowik TF, Bratzler DW, Kresowik RA, et al. Multistate improvement in process and outcomes of carotid endarterectomy. *J Vasc Surg*. 2004;39(2):372-80. PMID: 14743139.

95. Kresowik TF, Bratzler D, Karp HR, et al. Multistate utilization, processes, and outcomes of carotid endarterectomy. *J Vasc Surg*. 2001;33(2):227-34; discussion 34-5. PMID: 11174772.

96. Bratzler DW, Oehlert WH, Murray CK, et al. Carotid endarterectomy in Oklahoma Medicare beneficiaries: patient characteristics and outcomes. *J Okla State Med Assoc.* 1996;89(12):423-9. PMID: 8997882.

97. Cebul RD, Snow RJ, Pine R, et al. Indications, outcomes, and provider volumes for carotid endarterectomy. *JAMA.* 1998;279(16):1282-7. PMID: 9565009.

98. Halm EA, Tuhrim S, Wang JJ, et al. Risk factors for perioperative death and stroke after carotid endarterectomy: results of the new york carotid artery surgery study. *Stroke.* 2009;40(1):221-9. PMID: 18948605.

99. Halm EA, Chassin MR, Tuhrim S, et al. Revisiting the appropriateness of carotid endarterectomy. *Stroke.* 2003;34(6):1464-71. PMID: 12738896.

100. Rockman CB, Halm EA, Wang JJ, et al. Primary closure of the carotid artery is associated with poorer outcomes during carotid endarterectomy. *J Vasc Surg.* 2005;42(5):870-7. PMID: 16275440.

101. Halm EA, Hannan EL, Rojas M, et al. Clinical and operative predictors of outcomes of carotid endarterectomy. *J Vasc Surg.* 2005;42(3):420-8. PMID: 16171582.

102. Press MJ, Chassin MR, Wang J, et al. Predicting medical and surgical complications of carotid endarterectomy: comparing the risk indexes. *Arch Intern Med.* 2006;166(8):914-20. PMID: 16636219.

103. Karp HR, Flanders WD, Shipp CC, et al. Carotid endarterectomy among Medicare beneficiaries: a statewide evaluation of appropriateness and outcome. *Stroke.* 1998;29(1):46-52. PMID: 9445327.

104. Kresowik TF, Hemann RA, Grund SL, et al. Improving the outcomes of carotid endarterectomy: results of a statewide quality improvement project. *J Vasc Surg.* 2000;31(5):918-26. PMID: 10805882.

105. Hopkins LN, Roubin GS, Chakhtoura EY, et al. The Carotid Revascularization Endarterectomy versus Stenting Trial: credentialing of interventionalists and final results of lead-in phase. *J Stroke Cerebrovasc Dis.* 2010;19(2):153-62. PMID: 20189092.

106. Giacovelli JK, Egorova N, Dayal R, et al. Outcomes of carotid stenting compared with endarterectomy are equivalent in asymptomatic patients and inferior in symptomatic patients. *J Vasc Surg.* 2010;52(4):906-13, 13 e1-4. PMID: 20620010.

107. Vouyouka AG, Egorova NN, Sosunov EA, et al. Analysis of Florida and New York state hospital discharges suggests that carotid stenting in symptomatic women is associated with significant increase in mortality and perioperative morbidity compared with carotid endarterectomy. *J Vasc Surg.* 2012;56(2):334-42. PMID: 22583852.

108. Yuo TH, Degenholtz HS, Chaer RA, et al. Effect of hospital-level variation in the use of carotid artery stenting versus carotid endarterectomy on perioperative stroke and death in asymptomatic patients. *J Vasc Surg.* 2013;57(3):627-34. PMID: 23312937.

109. McPhee JT, Hill JS, Ciocca RG, et al. Carotid endarterectomy was performed with lower stroke and death rates than carotid artery stenting in the United States in 2003 and 2004. *J Vasc Surg.* 2007;46(6):1112-8. PMID: 18154987.

110. McPhee JT, Schanzer A, Messina LM, et al. Carotid artery stenting has increased rates of postprocedure stroke, death, and resource utilization than does carotid endarterectomy in the United States, 2005. *J Vasc Surg.* 2008;48(6):1442-50, 50 e1. PMID: 18829236.

111. Timaran CH, Veith FJ, Rosero EB, et al. Intracranial hemorrhage after carotid endarterectomy and carotid stenting in the United States in 2005. *J Vasc Surg.* 2009;49(3):623-8; discussion 8-9. PMID: 19268766.

112. Giles KA, Hamdan AD, Pomposelli FB, et al. Stroke and death after carotid endarterectomy and carotid artery stenting with and without high risk criteria. *J Vasc Surg.* 2010;52(6):1497-504. PMID: 20864299.

113. Young KC, Jahromi BS. Does current practice in the United States of carotid artery stent placement benefit asymptomatic octogenarians? *AJNR Am J Neuroradiol.* 2011;32(1):170-3. PMID: 20864521.

114. Woo K, Garg J, Hye RJ, et al. Contemporary results of carotid endarterectomy for asymptomatic carotid stenosis. *Stroke.* 2010;41(5):975-9. PMID: 20339122.

115. Garg J, Frankel DA, Dilley RB. Carotid endarterectomy in academic versus community hospitals: the national surgical quality improvement program data. *Ann Vasc Surg.* 2011;25(4):433-41. PMID: 21435832.

116. Wallaert JB, De Martino RR, Finlayson SR, et al. Carotid endarterectomy in asymptomatic patients with limited life expectancy. *Stroke.* 2012;43(7):1781-7. PMID: 22550053.

117. Fokkema M, Bensley RP, Lo RC, et al. In-hospital versus postdischarge adverse events following carotid endarterectomy. *J Vasc Surg.* 2013;57(6):1568-75, 75 e1-3. PMID: 23388394.

118. Horner RD, Oddone EZ, Stechuchak KM, et al. Racial variations in postoperative outcomes of carotid endarterectomy: evidence from the Veterans Affairs National Surgical Quality Improvement Program. Med Care. 2002;40(1 Suppl):I35-43. PMID: 11789630.

119. Samsa G, Oddone EZ, Horner R, et al. To what extent should quality of care decisions be based on health outcomes data? Application to carotid endarterectomy. *Stroke.* 2002;33(12):2944-9. PMID: 12468795.

120. Mercado N, Cohen DJ, Spertus JA, et al. Carotid artery stenting of a contralateral occlusion and in-hospital outcomes: results from the CARE (Carotid Artery Revascularization and Endarterectomy) registry. *JACC Cardiovasc Interv.* 2013;6(1):59-64. PMID: 23347862.

121. Rajamani K, Kennedy KF, Ruggiero NJ, et al. Outcomes of carotid endarterctomy in the elderly: A report from the care registry(registered trademark). *Stroke.* 2012;43(2).

122. Theiss W, Hermanek P, Mathias K, et al. Predictors of death and stroke after carotid angioplasty and stenting: a subgroup analysis of the Pro-CAS data. *Stroke.* 2008;39(8):2325-30. PMID: 18583556.

123. Palombo D, Lucertini G, Mambrini S, et al. Carotid endarterectomy: results of the Italian Vascular Registry. *J Cardiovasc Surg.* 2009;50(2):183-7. PMID: 19282808.

124. Micari A, Stabile E, Cremonesi A, et al. Carotid artery stenting in octogenarians using a proximal endovascular occlusion cerebral protection device: a multicenter registry. *Catheter Cardiovasc Interv.* 2010;76(1):9-15. PMID: 20578188.

125. Menyhei G, Bjorck M, Beiles B, et al. Outcome following carotid endarterectomy: lessons learned from a large international vascular registry. *Eur J Vasc Endovasc Surg.* 2011;41(6):735-40. PMID: 21450496.

126. Lindstrom D, Jonsson M, Formgren J, et al. Outcome after 7 years of carotid artery stenting and endarterectomy in Sweden - single centre and national results. *Eur J Vasc Endovasc Surg.* 2012;43(5):499-503. PMID: 22342694.

127. Sidawy AN, Zwolak RM, White RA, et al. Risk-adjusted 30-day outcomes of carotid stenting and endarterectomy: results from the SVS Vascular Registry. *J Vasc Surg.* 2009;49(1):71-9. PMID: 19028045.

128. Jim J, Rubin BG, Ricotta JJ, 2nd, et al. Society for Vascular Surgery (SVS) Vascular Registry evaluation of comparative effectiveness of carotid revascularization procedures stratified by Medicare age. *J Vasc Surg.* 2012;55(5):1313-20; discussion 21. PMID: 22459755.

129. Schermerhorn ML, Fokkema M, Goodney P, et al. The impact of Centers for Medicare and Medicaid Services high-risk criteria on outcome after carotid endarterectomy and carotid artery stenting in the SVS Vascular Registry. *J Vasc Surg.* 2013;57(5):1318-24. PMID: 23406712.

130. Lal BK, Meschia JF, Brott TG. CREST-2: guiding treatments for asymptomatic carotid disease. *Endovascular Today.* 2013(September):73-6.

131. Abbott AL. Medical (nonsurgical) intervention alone is now best for prevention of stroke associated with asymptomatic severe carotid stenosis: results of a systematic review and analysis. *Stroke.* 2009;40(10):e573-83. PMID: 19696421.

132. Brewer NT, Salz T, Lillie SE. Systematic review: the long-term effects of false-positive mammograms. *Ann Intern Med.* 2007;146(7):502-10. PMID: 17404352.

133. Hewlett J, Waisbren SE. A review of the psychosocial effects of false-positive results on parents and current communication practices in newborn screening. *J Inherit Metab Dis.* 2006;29(5):677-82. PMID: 16917730.

134. Carlsson S, Aus G, Wessman C, et al. Anxiety associated with prostate cancer screening with special reference to men with a positive screening test (elevated PSA) - Results from a prospective, population-based, randomised study. *Eur J Cancer.* 2007;43(14):2109-16. PMID: 17643983.

135. Esserman LJ, Thompson IM, Jr., Reid B. Overdiagnosis and overtreatment in cancer: an opportunity for improvement. *JAMA.* 2013;310(8):797-8. PMID: 23896967.

136. Welch HG, Black WC. Overdiagnosis in cancer. *J Natl Cancer Inst.* 2010;102(9):605-13. PMID: 20413742.

137. U.S. Preventive Services Task Force. Guide to Clinical Preventive Services. 2nd ed. Rockville, MD: Agency for Healthcare Research and Quality;1996.

138. Ratchford EV, Jin Z, Di Tullio MR, et al. Carotid bruit for detection of hemodynamically significant carotid stenosis: the Northern Manhattan Study. *Neurol Res.* 2009;31(7):748-52. PMID: 19133168.

139. Cournot M, Boccalon H, Cambou JP, et al. Accuracy of the screening physical examination to identify subclinical atherosclerosis and peripheral arterial disease in asymptomatic subjects. *J Vasc Surg.* 2007;46(6):1215-21. PMID: 18154997.

140. Johansson EP, Wester P. Carotid bruits as predictor for carotid stenoses detected by ultrasonography: an observational study. *BMC Neurol.* 2008;8:23. PMID: 18577216.

141. Cheng SW, Wu LL, Ting AC, et al. Screening for asymptomatic carotid stenosis in patients with peripheral vascular disease: a prospective study and risk factor analysis. *Cardiovasc Surg.* 1999;7(3):303-9. PMID: 10386747.

142. Paraskevas KI, Mikhailidis DP, Liapis CD, et al. Critique of the Carotid Revascularization Endarterectomy versus Stenting Trial (CREST): flaws in CREST and its interpretation. *Eur J Vasc Endovasc Surg.* 2013;45(6):539-45. PMID: 23602856.

143.   Rothwell PM. Carotid stenting: more risky than endarterectomy and often no better than medical treatment alone. *Lancet*. 2010;375(9719):957-9. PMID: 20304225.

144.   Raman G, Kitsios GD, Moorthy D, et al. Management of Asymptomatic Carotid Stenosis: Technology Assessment Report. Rockville, MD: Agency for Healthcare Research and Quality; 2012.

145.   Helfand M, Buckley DI, Freeman M, et al. Emerging risk factors for coronary heart disease: a summary of systematic reviews conducted for the U.S. Preventive Services Task Force. *Ann Intern Med*. 2009;151(7):496-507. PMID: 19805772.

146.   Takaya N, Yuan C, Chu B, et al. Association between carotid plaque characteristics and subsequent ischemic cerebrovascular events: a prospective assessment with MRI—initial results. *Stroke*. 2006;37(3):818-23. PMID: 16469957.

147.   King A, Shipley M, Markus H. Optimizing protocols for risk prediction in asymptomatic carotid stenosis using embolic signal detection: the Asymptomatic Carotid Emboli Study. *Stroke*. 2011;42(10):2819-24. PMID: 21852607.

148.   Hoke M, Speidl W, Schillinger M, et al. Polymorphism of the complement 5 gene and cardiovascular outcome in patients with atherosclerosis. *Eur J Clin Invest*. 2012;42(9):921-6. PMID: 22452399.

149.   Molloy J, Markus HS. Asymptomatic embolization predicts stroke and TIA risk in patients with carotid artery stenosis. *Stroke*. 1999;30(7):1440-3. PMID: 10390320.

150.   Spence JD, Tamayo A, Lownie SP, et al. Absence of microemboli on transcranial Doppler identifies low-risk patients with asymptomatic carotid stenosis. *Stroke*. 2005;36(11):2373-8. PMID: 16224084.

151.   Brott TG, Halperin JL, Abbara S, et al. 2011 ASA/ACCF/AHA/AANN/AANS/ACR/ASNR/CNS/SAIP/SCAI/SIR/SNIS/SVM/SVS guideline on the management of patients with extracranial carotid and vertebral artery disease. *Stroke*. 2011;42(8):e464-540. PMID: 21282493.

152.   Ricotta JJ, Aburahma A, Ascher E, et al. Updated Society for Vascular Surgery guidelines for management of extracranial carotid disease. *J Vasc Surg*. 2011;54(3):e1-31. PMID: 21889701.

Figure 1. Analytic Framework

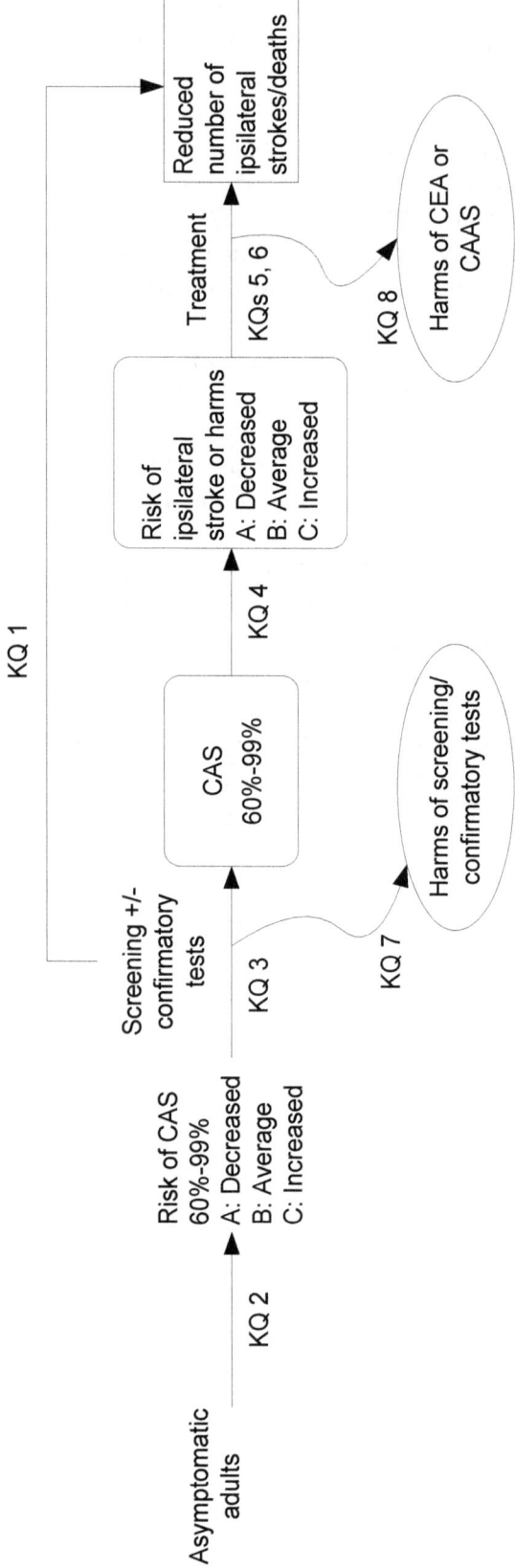

Abbreviations: CAS = carotid artery stenosis; CAAS = carotid angioplasty and stenting; CEA = carotid endarterectomy; KQ = key question.

Figure 2. Summary of Evidence Search and Selection

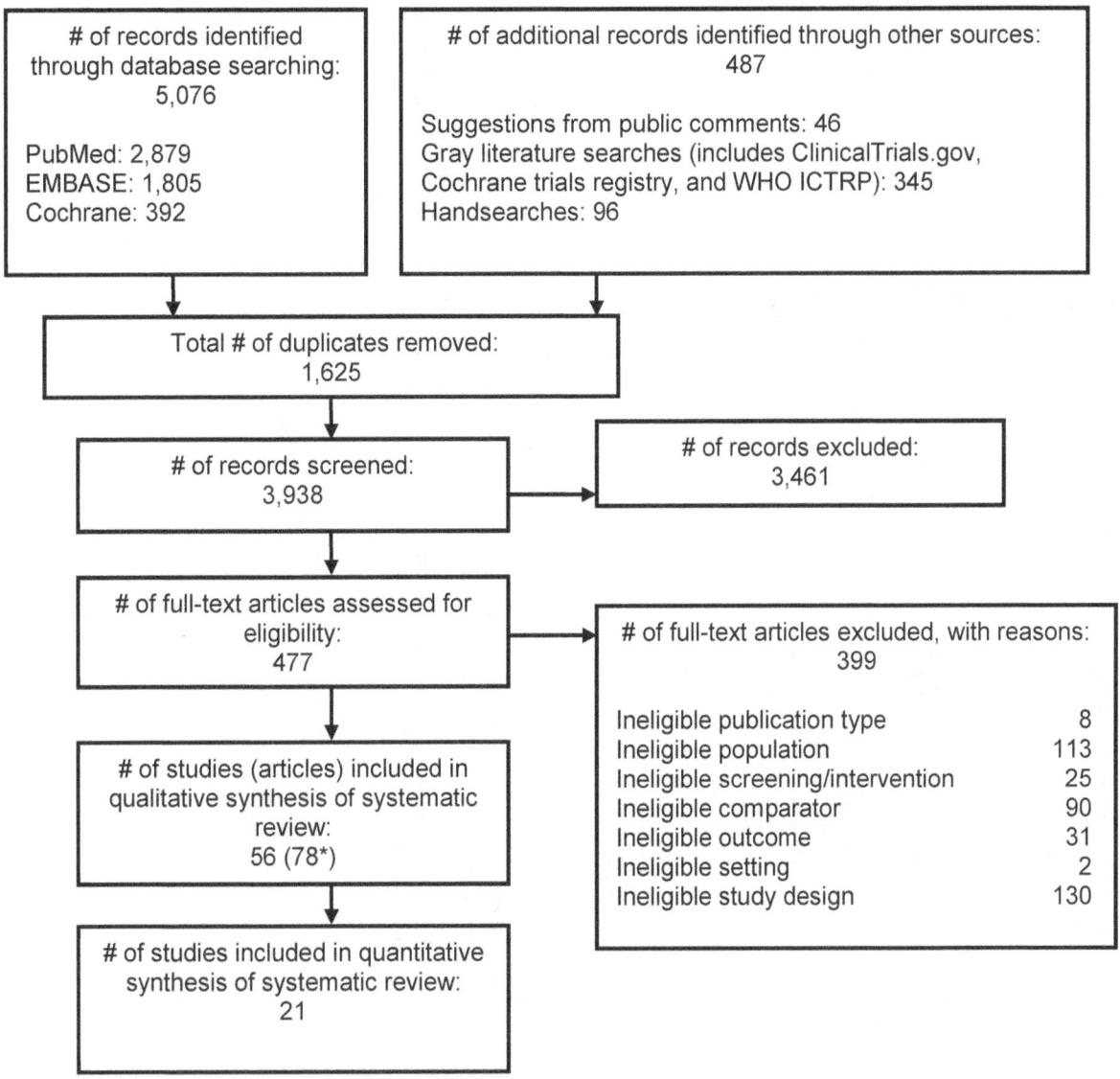

* Includes methods papers for included trials.

Abbreviation: WHO ICTRP = World Health Organization International Clinical Trials Registry Platform.

Table 1. Studies Attempting to Externally Validate Risk Stratification Tools to Distinguish Persons Who Are More or Less Likely to Have CAS

Author, Year Country	Derivation Cohort (N)	External Validation Cohort (N)	Predicted Outcome	Model Components[a]	% With Actual CAS	% With CAS by Risk Score	Model Assessment: AUROC C-statistic	Model Assessment: Other	% Studied in Effectiveness or CE Studies	Quality
Suri, 2008 United States	Jacobowitz, 2003 (394) Mean age: 71.3 y Male: 32% White: 86% DM: NR HTN: 64% HChol: 45% Sm: 8% CAD: 17.3% Qureshi, 2001 (887) Mean age: 66 y Male: 31% White: NR DM: 7% HTN: 53% HChol: 15% Sm: 11% CAD: 11%	(5,795) Mean age: 72 y Male: 42% White: 84% DM: NR HTN: 54% HChol: 57% Sm: 11% CAD: 8%	CAS ≥50% CAS ≥75%	Jacobowitz[a]: Sm, HChol, HTN, CAD Qureshi[b]: Age >65 y, Sm, HChol, CAD	Suri, full cohort: ≥50%: 4.2 50%-74%: 3.2 ≥75%: 1.0 75%-99%: 0.7 Jacobowitz model: >50%: 9.6 >75%: NR Qureshi model: >60%: 18.0 (full sample) >75%: NR	Jacobowitz model, ≥50% by score: 1: 2.9 2: 5.1 3: 8.1 4: 20.7 ≥75% by score: 1: 0.7 2: 1.1 3: 2.1 4: 3.4 Qureshi model, ≥50% by score: 1: 4.0 2: 5.3 3: 7.4 4: 18.9 ≥75% by score: 1: 0.8 2: 1.8 3: 2.1 4: 2.7	For CAS ≥50%: Jacobowitz model: 0.60 (95% CI, 0.56 to 0.64) Qureshi model: 0.56 (95% CI, 0.53 to 0.60) For CAS ≥75%: Jacobowitz model: 0.60 (95% CI, 0.52 to 0.68) Qureshi model: 0.58 (95% CI, 0.50 to 0.67)	LR for ≥50% CAS: Jacobowitz: Score 4: 6 Qureshi[c] Score 4: 5.4 LR for ≥75% CAS: Jacobowitz: Score 4: 3.7 Qureshi[c] Score 4: 2.9 HL chi square: NA Net reclassification: NA	NR	Fair for attempted external validation of Jacobowitz model Poor for Qureshi model

[a] Jacobowitz risk score: 1 point for each risk factor (range, 0–4); predicts stenosis >50%.
[b] Qureshi risk score: 1 point for smoking, 2 points for CAD, 1 point for HChol, 4 points for age >65 years; predicts stenosis >60%.
[c] Age not used in risk calculation for validation because all participants were older than age 65 years.

Abbreviations: AUROC = area under receiver operating characteristic; CAS = carotid artery stenosis; CAD = coronary artery disease; CE = comparative effectiveness; DM = diabetes mellitus; Hchol = hypercholesterolemia; HTN = hypertension; LR = likelihood ratio; M = male; NA = not applicable; N = sample size; NR = not reported; Sm = smoker; W = white.

Table 2. Characteristics of Included Randomized, Controlled Trials of CEA Compared With Medical Management for Asymptomatic CAS

Study, year	N	Country	Source of Patients	Medical Management Description	Followup	Age	% White	% Male	% DM % HTN % HChol % Sm % CAD	% Prior contralateral CEA	% Contralateral occlusion	% Contralateral TIA/stroke	Pre-randomization evaluation & required stenosis	Quality
ACAS, 1995	1,662	United States & Canada	U/S labs, practitioners who found bruits or carotid stenosis during evaluation for peripheral vascular surgery or contralateral CEA	All patients received 325 mg of regular or enteric-coated aspirin daily. Also had risk factor discussion and modification at randomization, subsequent interviews, and telephone followup	2.7 y	67 y	95	66	23 64 NR 26 69	20	9	25	U/S or angiogram: ≥60%	Good for the 2.7-y data that was based on actual events; Fair for the 5-y estimates; only 9% had followup to 5 y
ACST, 2004 and 2010	3,120	30 countries (most in Europe; also included Russia, Israel, and 16 subjects from United States)	Medical and surgical clinics	Left to discretion of clinicians, usually included antiplatelet and antihypertensive therapy; in later years of the trial, lipid-lowering therapy was common[a]	Median in survivors: 9 y (IQR, 6 to 11)[b]	68 y	NR	66	20 65 27 (≥250 mg/dL) NR Non-DM CAD: 27	24	9	NR	U/S: ≥60%	Fair
VACS, 1993	444	United States	11 VAMCs, patients scheduled for surgery who had asymptomatic stenoses, patients with unilateral symptomatic lesions found to have contralateral asymptomatic stenosis on arteriography, and patients with incidental cervical bruits and positive noninvasive screening tests	650 mg aspirin BID, reduced to 325 mg daily if not tolerated	4 y	65 y	87	100	27-30 63-64 NR 49-52 Hx of MI: 25-28	NR	NR	32	Angiogram: ≥50%	Good

[a]At study entry, 17% of subjects randomized in 1993 to 1996 were on lipid-lowering therapy; it increased to 58% in 2000 to 2003. At the last followup in 2002 to 2003, >90% of the survivors were on antiplatelet therapy, 81% were on antihypertensives, and 70% were on lipid-lowering therapy. At followup in 2002 or 2003, mean blood pressure was 148/79 mm Hg in both groups.
[b]Followup to death or at least year 3 is 98% complete (3,062/3,120).

Abbreviations: ACAS = Asymptomatic Carotid Atherosclerosis Study; ACST = Asymptomatic Carotid Surgery Trial; CAD = coronary artery disease; CEA = carotid endarterectomy; DM = diabetes mellitus; Hchol = hypercholesterolemia; HTN = hypertension; N = sample size; PVD = peripheral vascular disease; Sm = smoker; TIA = transient ischemic attack; U/S = ultrasound; VACS = Veterans' Affairs Cooperative Study; VAMC = Veterans Administration Medical Center.

Table 3. Main Results of Randomized, Controlled Trials of CEA Compared With Medical Management for Asymptomatic CAS

Study, year	Require preoperative angiogram?	Angiogram complication rate	Perioperative (30-d) stroke or death	Perioperative (30-d) nonfatal MI	Rate of perioperative stroke/death & any subsequent stroke (95% CI)	Rate of perioperative stroke/death & subsequent ipsilateral stroke (95% CI)	All-cause mortality (# of deaths)	Any stroke or death	QOL or functional status
ACAS, 1995	Yes	1.2% (5 patients had CVAs, 1 of whom died; 414 had angiograms)	2.7%[a] Sex: W: 3.6% M: 1.7% p=0.12	NR	5-y estimate: MM: 17.5% CEA: 12.4% RRR: 29% (-5% to 52%) ARR: 5.1% Observed events, median 2.7-y followup: MM: 10.3% CEA: 7.3% ARR: 3% By age, sex, race, ethnicity: NR	5-y estimate: MM: 11% (NR) CEA: 5.1% (NR) RRR: 53% (22% to 72%) ARR: 5.9% (NR) Observed events, median 2.7-y followup: MM: 6.2% CEA: 4% ARR: 2.2% 5-y RRR: Sex W: 17% (-96% to 65%) M: 66% (36% to 82%) Age <68 y: 60% (11% to 82%) ≥68 y: 43% (-7% to 70%)	MM: 89 CEA: 83	5-y estimate: MM: 31.9% CEA: 25.6% RRR: 20% (-2% to 37%) ARR: 6.3% Observed events, median 2.7-y followup: MM: 18.6% CEA: 15.4% ARR: 3.2%	NR
ACST, 2004 and 2010	No	NA	2.9% (2.1 to 3.8)[b] No significant difference for subgroups of age, sex, or extent of stenosis[c]	0.7%	10-y estimate: MM: 13.1% CEA: 9.2% RR: 0.70 (0.57 to 0.86) ARR: 3.9% By age, sex, race, ethnicity: NR[d]	MM: 6.9% CEA: 5.3% RR: 0.76 (0.57 to 1.00) ARR: 1.6%	MM: 570 CEA: 610[e]	MM: 49.4% CEA: 47.2% RR: 0.95 (0.89 to 1.03)	Proportion of nonperioperative strokes that were disabling or fatal: 57.8% (166/287). Reduction in disabling or fatal nonperioperative stroke: 0.61 (95% CI, 0.41 to 0.92)
VACS, 1993	Yes	0.4% (3 nonfatal strokes/714 angiograms)	4.7%[f] By age, sex, race, ethnicity: NR	1.9% (4/211)	MM: 12.9% CEA: 10.4% RR: 0.81 (0.48 to 1.36) ARR: 2.5% By age, sex, race, ethnicity: NR	MM: 10.3% CEA: 6.6% RR: 0.64 (0.34 to 1.21) ARR: 3.7%[g]	MM: 78 CEA: 70	MM: 44.2% CEA: 41.2% RR: 0.92 (0.69 to 1.22)	Mean stroke severity score[h]: MM: 4.1 CEA: 3.6 P: NS

[a]During the perioperative period, 2.3% of surgical patients (n=19) had a stroke or died (95% CI, 1.28 to 3.32) compared with 0.4% of patients in the medical group (95% CI, 0.0% to 0.8%). It was estimated that if all 724 patients receiving CEA had undergone arteriography as part of the ACAS (some had an angiogram in the 60 days prior to the study) that 2.7% of surgical patients would have had stroke or death from the procedure.

[b]2.9% (44 of 1,532 CEAs performed) was the rate of perioperative stroke or death for the immediate CEA group; when including the delayed group that underwent CEA, the rate was 3.0% (95% CI, 2.4 to 3.9).

[c]Data not shown; reported in text only in the 10-year followup publication of ACST. The 5-year followup publication of ACST reported rates of 3.6% for women, 2.5% for men, 2.6% for those age <65 years, 2.6% for those ages 65 to 74 years, and 3.7% for those age ≥75 years; these data are from an online table referenced in the initial results paper from ACST and do not include all 1,532 CEAs reported in the later publication. The denominator was 1,405 CEAs performed in the immediate CEA group.

[d]Not reported by subgroups for this outcome, but reported for some other outcomes. First nonperioperative stroke, by sex: W, 0.57 (95% CI, 0.34 to 0.97); M, 0.52 (95% CI, 0.36 to 0.75). First nonperioperative stroke, by age: <65 years at entry, 0.46 (95% CI, 0.26 to 0.82); 65 to 74 years at entry, 0.48 (95% CI, 0.31 to 0.75); ≥75 years at entry, 0.81 (95% CI, 0.43 to 1.51).

[e]Obtained from online Appendix Table 2A. Cause-specific number of deaths within 10 years for MM (deferral) vs. immediate CEA: perioperative (i.e., after CEA), 3 vs. 17 (p=0.002); nonperioperative stroke, 68 vs. 39 (p=0.006); vascular, 267 vs. 298 (p=0.15); neoplastic, 101 vs. 111 (p=0.44); other/unknown, 131 vs. 145 (p=0.33).

Table 3. Main Results of Randomized, Controlled Trials of CEA Compared With Medical Management for Asymptomatic CAS

[f]30-day operative mortality was 1.9% (4/211), with 3 deaths from MI and 1 from MI followed by stroke. During the perioperative period, 4.7% of surgical patients had a stroke or died, when including the complications of arteriography, compared with 1 death due to suicide (0.4%), 1 stroke (0.4%), and 1 TIA (0.4%) in the medical group.

[g]Incidence of all ipsilateral neurologic events (TIA, transient monocular blindness, fatal stroke, and nonfatal stroke): MM, 48 (20.6%) vs. CEA, 17 (8%); RR, 0.38 (95% CI, 0.22 to 0.67). Incidence of ipsilateral stroke (fatal and nonfatal): MM, 22 (9.4%) vs. 10 (4.7%); 95% CI, NR.

[h]1 to 11 scale: 1 to 3 = no impairment, 4 = minor impairment, ≥5 = major impairment in at least one domain of functioning.

Abbreviations: ACAS = Asymptomatic Carotid Atherosclerosis Study; ACST = Asymptomatic Carotid Surgery Trial; ARR = absolute risk reduction; CEA = carotid endarterectomy; CI = confidence interval; CVA = cerebrovascular accident; M = men; MI = myocardial infarction; MM = medical management; NA = not applicable; NR = not reported; NS = not significant; RR = relative risk; RRR = relative risk reduction; W = women.

Table 4. Characteristics of Additional Studies Rated as Good or Fair Quality and Reporting Rates of Periprocedural Complications of CEA or CAAS for Adults With Asymptomatic CAS

Study, Year	Design Study Period	Procedure N Total (N Asymp)	Setting and Source Population	Sample Selection Criteria	Sample Subjects' Characteristics[a]	Threats to Internal and External Validity	Quality
Cohort studies							
Bratzler, 1996	Cohort study 1/1993-12/1994	CEA 813 (347); 774 patients	Oklahoma Medicare beneficiaries, 8 hospitals	Medicare claims used to identify all CEA cases. Asymptomatic defined as no prior TIA or stroke in the distribution of the operated carotid artery.	Median Age: 73 y White: NR Female: NR DM: 26% CAD: 67% COPD: 20% HF: 10% HTN: 71% Smoker: 26% Stenosis: 96% >60% CAS Prior contralateral CEA: NR Contralateral occlusion: NR Contralateral TIA/stroke: NR	May have missed nonfatal neurologic events occurring after discharge that did not result in another hospitalization; no comprehensive exam by neurologist for outcome assessment; definition of symptomatic CAS required documentation of past TIA or stroke in the distribution of the carotid being operated on.	Fair
Cebul, 1998	Cohort study 7/1993-6/1994	CEA 678 (167)	Ohio non-HMO Medicare beneficiaries, 115 hospitals and at least 478 surgeons	Medicare part A claims used to identify all non-HMO Medicare beneficiaries who underwent CEA; random sample of the 4120 CEAs performed. Asymptomatic if no record of any neurologic symptoms or signs; categorized as nonspecific symptoms if had nonlateralizing symptoms or signs (e.g., dizziness, dementia)	Mean Age: 73 y White: 94% Female: 46% DM: 26% CAD: NR COPD: 15% HF: 9% HTN: 71% Smoker: 31% Stenosis: NR Prior contralateral CEA: NR Contralateral occlusion: NR Contralateral TIA/stroke: NR	May have missed nonfatal neurologic events occurring after discharge that did not result in another hospitalization; no comprehensive exam by neurologist for outcome assessment; interrater reliability for determining indication for surgery (TIA, stroke, asymptomatic or nonspecific symptoms) of 77% (kappa, 0.69).	Fair

Table 4. Characteristics of Additional Studies Rated as Good or Fair Quality and Reporting Rates of Periprocedural Complications of CEA or CAAS for Adults With Asymptomatic CAS

Study, Year	Design Study Period	Procedure N Total (N Asymp)	Setting and Source Population	Sample Selection Criteria	Sample Subjects' Characteristics[a]	Threats to Internal and External Validity	Quality
Giacovelli, 2010	Cohort study 2005-2007	CEA + CAAS 47,752 total CAAS+CEA (42,236) 4,919 (4,353) used in the matched propensity analysis comparing CAAS and CEA	New York and California state hospital discharge databases	ICD-9 codes to identify patients who had CAAS or CEA. Uses "present on admission" (POA) flag in discharge diagnoses to identify symptom status.	Mean Age:[b] CEA: 73 y; CAAS: 71 y White: CEA: 86%; CAAS: 77% Female: CEA: 43%; CAAS: 39% DM: CEA: 27%; CAAS: 30% CAD/HF: CEA: 44%; CAAS: 57% COPD: CEA: 14%; CAAS: 13% HTN: CEA: 71%; CAAS: 74% Smoker: NR Stenosis: NR Prior contralateral CEA: NR Contralateral occlusion: NR Contralateral TIA/stroke: NR	Used present on admission designations to determine symptom status at baseline; used ICD-9 codes only for outcome ascertainment; no supplementation with review of medical records; in-hospital outcomes only.	Fair
Giles, 2010	Cohort study 10/2004-12/2007	CEA + CAAS 538,958 (52,937) CAAS: 56,564 (49,126) CEA: 482,394 (436,895)	NIS database[c]	ICD-9 codes from NIS database. Patients with symptomatic carotid stenosis were identified by ICD-9 diagnosis codes of TIA, amaurosis fugax, or stroke. Patients also classified as CMS high risk based on prespecified criteria.	Mean Age: CEA: 71 y; CAAS: 70 y White: NR Female: CEA: 43%; CAAS: 40% DM: NR CAD (Previous MI): CEA: 11%; CAAS: 10% COPD: CEA: 22%; CAAS: 19% HF: CEA: 7%; CAAS: 11% HTN: NR Smoker: NR Stenosis: NR Prior contralateral CEA: NR Contralateral occlusion: NR Contralateral TIA/stroke: NR	Used ICD-9 codes only for outcome ascertainment; no supplementation with review of medical records; in-hospital outcomes only; potential for bias due to misclassification of symptom status and whether stroke was the indication or a perioperative harm.	Fair

Table 4. Characteristics of Additional Studies Rated as Good or Fair Quality and Reporting Rates of Periprocedural Complications of CEA or CAAS for Adults With Asymptomatic CAS

Study, Year	Design Study Period	Procedure N Total (N Asymp)	Setting and Source Population	Sample Selection Criteria	Sample Subjects' Characteristics[a]	Threats to Internal and External Validity	Quality
Halm, 2003; Rockma, 2005; Halm, 2005; Press, 2006	Cohort study 1/1997-12/1998	CEA 2,124 (1,413) (N varies slightly across publications)	6 hospitals in New York (4 university and 2 community hospitals); 67 surgeons	Used administrative databases from 6 hospitals; consecutive CEAs (identified by ICD-9 codes). Indication for surgery based on acuity of the presenting neurologic symptoms in the 12 months before surgery (stroke-in-evolution, stroke, carotid TIA, asymptomatic, etc.).	Mean Age: 72 y White: 87% Female: 43% DM: 29% CAD: 55% COPD: 9% HF: 8% HTN: 73% Smoker: NR% Stenosis: 90.1% had 70%-99% CAS: Prior contralateral CEA: NR Contralateral occlusion: 6% Contralateral TIA/stroke: NR	May have missed readmissions to other hospitals (only included readmissions to the index hospital); data from 1 region of New York; no comprehensive exam by neurologist for outcome assessment.	Fair
Halm, 2007; Halm, 2009	Cohort study (NYCAS) 1/1998-6/1999	CEA 9,588 (6,932)	New York state Medicare beneficiaries; 166 hospitals; 488 surgeons	Any NY state Medicare claims for CEA and NY state hospital discharge database.	Mean Age: 75 y White: 93% Female: 44% DM: 30% CAD: 62% COPD: 19% HF: 10% HTN: 79% Smoker: NR Stenosis: 94% with 70%-99%; 1% with 100% occlusion; 2.9% with 60%-69% Prior contralateral CEA: NR Contralateral occlusion: 5% with 100%; 24% with 70%-99%; 5% with 60%-69% Contralateral TIA/stroke: NR	May have missed nonfatal neurologic events occurring after discharge that did not result in another hospitalization; no comprehensive exam by neurologist for outcome assessment. Data abstractors had to pass a series of quality assurances and interrater reliability tests. Data reported had kappa from 0.60 to 1.0.	Fair

Table 4. Characteristics of Additional Studies Rated as Good or Fair Quality and Reporting Rates of Periprocedural Complications of CEA or CAAS for Adults With Asymptomatic CAS

Study, Year	Design Study Period	Procedure N Total (N Asymp)	Setting and Source Population	Sample Selection Criteria	Sample Subjects' Characteristics[a]	Threats to Internal and External Validity	Quality
Hopkins, 2010	Cohort study (lead-in/credentialing phase of CREST) 11/2000-4/2008	CAAS 1,565 (1,151)	Lead-in case data were reviewed prospectively for 427 potential interventionalists	Asymptomatic subjects had to have >70% stenosis by angiography. Ascertainment of symptom status is unclear; cases were submitted by potential interventionalists to a multidisciplinary committee for review.	Mean Age: 70 y White: 88% Female: 37% DM: 33% CAD: 24% with previous CABG COPD: NR HF: NR HTN: 84% Smoker: 18% Stenosis: 79% Prior contralateral CEA: NR Contralateral occlusion: NR Contralateral TIA/stroke:NR	Unclear whether cases are representative of the source population.	Fair
Karp, 1998	Cohort study 1/1993-12/1993	CEA 1,945 (1,002)	Georgia Medicare beneficiaries	Georgia Medicare claims; ICD-9 codes used to identify patients who underwent CEA. Asymptomatic defined following ACAS (absence of symptoms in distribution of the operated carotid artery).	Mean Age: 72 y White: 91% Female: 47% DM: 20% CAD: NR COPD: 24% HF: 8% HTN: NR Smoker: NR Stenosis: 22% had 56%-75%; 70% had >75% Prior contralateral CEA: NR Contralateral occlusion: NR Contralateral TIA/stroke: NR	May have missed nonfatal neurologic events occurring after discharge that did not result in another hospitalization; no comprehensive exam by neurologist for outcome assessment.	Fair
Kresowik, 2000	Cohort study 1/1994-12/1994 and 6/1995-5/1996	CEA 2,063 CEAs (671 CEAs; 1994 only: 159)	Iowa Medicare beneficiaries, 30 hospitals; 79 surgeons	Claims for CEA (ICD-9) from Medicare Provider Analysis and Review (MEDPAR) Part A claims; Part B files for CPT codes also used. Considered asymptomatic if no history prior to CEA of CV symptoms or events in either the anterior or posterior circulations.	Median Age: 74 y White: NR Female: 40%-41% DM: NR CAD: NR COPD: NR HF: NR HTN: NR Smoker: NR Stenosis: NR Prior contralateral CEA: NR Contralateral occlusion: NR Contralateral TIA/stroke: NR	May have missed nonfatal neurologic events occurring after discharge that did not result in another hospitalization; no comprehensive exam by neurologist for outcome assessment.	Fair

Table 4. Characteristics of Additional Studies Rated as Good or Fair Quality and Reporting Rates of Periprocedural Complications of CEA or CAAS for Adults With Asymptomatic CAS

Study, Year	Design Study Period	Procedure N Total (N Asymp)	Setting and Source Population	Sample Selection Criteria	Sample Subjects' Characteristics[a]	Threats to Internal and External Validity	Quality
Kresowik, 2001	Cohort study 6/1995–5/1996	CEA 10,561 (3,891); 10,030 patients	Medicare beneficiaries from 10 US states[d]	Used ICD-9 code for CEA among Medicare Provider Analysis and Review (MEDPAR) Part A claims. Considered asymptomatic if no history prior to CEA of CV symptoms or events in either the anterior or posterior circulations.	Mean age: 74 y White: NR Female: 43% DM: NR CAD: NR COPD: NR HF: NR HTN: NR Smoker: NR Stenosis: NR Prior contralateral CEA: NR Contralateral occlusion: NR Contralateral TIA/stroke: NR	May have missed nonfatal neurologic events occurring after discharge that did not result in another hospitalization; no comprehensive exam by neurologist for outcome assessment.	Fair
Kresowik, 2004	Cohort study 6/1995–5/1996 and 6/1998–5/1999	CEA 19,690 (1995-1996: 3,891; 1998-1999: 4,093)	Medicare beneficiaries from 10 US states[d]	ICD-9 code for CEA among Medicare Provider Analysis and Review (MEDPAR) Part A claims. Considered asymptomatic if there was no history prior to CEA of CV symptoms or events in the anterior or posterior circulations.	Median Age: 74 y White: NR Female: 43%–44% DM: NR CAD: NR COPD: NR HF: NR HTN: NR Smoker: NR Stenosis: NR Prior contralateral CEA: NR Contralateral occlusion: NR Contralateral TIA/stroke: NR	May have missed nonfatal neurologic events occurring after discharge that did not result in another hospitalization; no comprehensive exam by neurologist for outcome assessment.	Fair

Table 4. Characteristics of Additional Studies Rated as Good or Fair Quality and Reporting Rates of Periprocedural Complications of CEA or CAAS for Adults With Asymptomatic CAS

Study, Year	Design Study Period	Procedure N Total (N Asymp)	Setting and Source Population	Sample Selection Criteria	Sample Subjects' Characteristics[a]	Threats to Internal and External Validity	Quality
McPhee, 2007	Cohort study 1/2003-12/2004	CEA + CAAS 259,080 CEAs/CAASs (238,389 CEAs/ CAASs) 245,045 CEAs (226,111 CEAs) 14,035 CAASs (12,278 CAASs)	NIS (Nationwide Inpatient Sample)[c]	ICD-9 codes from NIS database	Mean Age: CEA: 71 y; CAAS: 71 y Median Age: CEA: 72 y; CAAS: 72 y White: NR Female: CEA: 43%; CAAS: 41% DM: CEA: 25%; CAAS: 26% CAD/MI: CEA: 12%; CAAS: 12% COPD: CEA: 19%; CAAS: 15% HF: CEA: 6%; CAAS: 9% HTN: CEA: 71%; CAAS: 67% Smoker: NR Stenosis: NR Prior contralateral CEA: NR Contralateral occlusion: NR Contralateral TIA/stroke: NR	Before 10/2004 no specific CAAS ICD-9 code existed, so required 2-step method to identify CAAS procedures with potential for misclassification. Used ICD-9 codes only for outcome ascertainment; no supplementation with review of medical records; in-hospital outcomes only; potential for bias due to misclassification of symptom status and whether stroke was the indication or a perioperative harm.	Fair
McPhee, 2008	Cohort study 2005	CEA + CAAS 135,701 (122,986) CEA: 122,786 (111,684) CAAS: 12,914 (11,302)	NIS database[c]	ICD-9 codes from NIS database	Mean Age:[b] CEA: 71; CAAS: 72 White: NR Female: CEA: 43%; CAAS: 37% DM: CEA: 27%; CAAS: 27% CAD/MI: CEA: 11%; CAAS: 12% COPD: CEA: 21%; CAAS: 18% HF: CEA: 7%; CAAS: 11% HTN: CEA: 72%; CAAS: 66% Smoker: NR Stenosis: NR Prior contralateral CEA: NR Contralateral occlusion: NR Contralateral TIA/stroke: NR	Used ICD-9 codes only for outcome ascertainment; no supplementation with review of medical records; in-hospital outcomes only; potential for bias due to misclassification of symptom status and whether stroke was the indication or a perioperative harm.	Fair

Table 4. Characteristics of Additional Studies Rated as Good or Fair Quality and Reporting Rates of Periprocedural Complications of CEA or CAAS for Adults With Asymptomatic CAS

Study, Year	Design Study Period	Procedure N Total (N Asymp)	Setting and Source Population	Sample Selection Criteria	Sample Subjects' Characteristics[a]	Threats to Internal and External Validity	Quality
Timaran, 2009	Cohort study 2005	CEA + CAAS CAAS:13,093 (11,836) CEA:122,984 (113,514)	NIS database[c]	ICD-9 codes from NIS database	Median Age: CEA: 72 y; CAAS: 72 y White: NR Female: CEA: 43%; CAAS: 38% DM: CEA: 29%; CAAS: 28% Previous MI: CEA: 12%; CAAS: 11% COPD: CEA: 21%; CAAS: 18% HF: CEA: 8%; CAAS: 12% HTN: CEA: 76%; CAAS: 69% Smoker: NR Stenosis: NR Prior contralateral CEA: NR Contralateral occlusion: NR Contralateral TIA/stroke: NR	Used ICD-9 codes only for outcome ascertainment; no supplementation with review of medical records; in-hospital outcomes only; potential for bias due to misclassification of symptom status and whether stroke was the indication or a perioperative harm.	Fair
Vouyouka, 2012	Cohort study 2007-2009	CEA + CAAS 20,613 CEAs/ CAASs (18,519) CEA: 18,320 (16,576) CAAS: 2,263 (1,943)	New York and Florida state discharge databases to identify women who underwent CEA or CAAS	ICD-9 codes to identify patients who had CAAS or CEA. Uses POA flag in discharge diagnoses to identify symptom status.	Mean Age:[b] 72 y White: 90% Female: 100% DM: 30% CAD: 37% COPD: 2% HF: 6% HTN: 80% Smoker: NR Stenosis: NR Prior contralateral CEA: NR Contralateral occlusion: NR Contralateral TIA/stroke: NR	Used present on admission designations to determine symptom status at baseline; used ICD-9 codes only for outcome ascertainment; no supplementation with review of medical records; in-hospital outcomes only.	Fair

Table 4. Characteristics of Additional Studies Rated as Good or Fair Quality and Reporting Rates of Periprocedural Complications of CEA or CAAS for Adults With Asymptomatic CAS

Study, Year	Design Study Period	Procedure N Total (N Asymp)	Setting and Source Population	Sample Selection Criteria	Sample Subjects' Characteristics[a]	Threats to Internal and External Validity	Quality
Young, 2011	Cohort study 2006-2007	CEA + CAAS 249,592 (all asymptomatic) CAAS: 31,197 (all) CEA: 218,395 (all)	NIS database[c]	ICD-9 codes from NIS database. Asymptomatic precerebral stenosis codes as indication for CAS/CEA, excluding TIA as indication for CAAS/CEA. Also stratified patients by age <80 years and ≥80 years.	Mean Age: 71 y; CEA: 71 y; CAAS: 71 y White: 66%; CEA: 65%; CAAS: 68% Female: 43%; CEA: 43%; CAAS: 40% DM: 31%; CEA: 31%; CAAS: 30% CAD (previous MI): 50%; CEA: 49%; CAAS: 57% COPD: 18%; CEA: 19%; CAAS: 18% HF: 8%; CEA: 7%; CAAS: 12% HTN: 79%; CEA: 79%; CAAS: 75% Smoker: 34%; CEA: 35%; CAAS: 27% Stenosis: NR Prior contralateral CEA: NR Contralateral stenosis: 17%; CEA: 17%; CAAS: 20% Contralateral occlusion: NR Contralateral TIA/stroke: NR	Used ICD-9 codes only for outcome ascertainment; no supplementation with review of medical records; in-hospital outcomes only; potential for bias due to misclassification of symptom status and whether stroke was the indication or a perioperative harm.	Fair

Table 4. Characteristics of Additional Studies Rated as Good or Fair Quality and Reporting Rates of Periprocedural Complications of CEA or CAAS for Adults With Asymptomatic CAS

Study, Year	Design Study Period	Procedure N Total (N Asymp)	Setting and Source Population	Sample Selection Criteria	Sample Subjects' Characteristics[a]	Threats to Internal and External Validity	Quality
Yuo, 2013	Cohort study 2005-2009	CEA + CAAS 30,317 (all asymptomatic) CAAS: 3,476 (all) CEA: 26,841 (all)	California hospital discharge data	ICD-9 codes to identify cerebral revascularization procedures. Symptom status determined by presence of admission or diagnosis codes for hemispheric cerebral ischemia or ophthalmic artery occlusion or embolism.	Age >70 y: CEA: 66%; CAAS: 62% White: CEA: 90%; CAAS: 83% Female: CEA: 43%; CAAS: 44% DM, complicated: CEA: 5%; CAAS: 4% Previous MI: NR COPD: CEA: 20%; CAAS: 17% HF: CEA: 8%; CAAS: 11% HTN, complicated: CEA: 10%; CAAS: 11% Smoker: NR Stenosis: NR Prior contralateral CEA: NR Contralateral occlusion: NR Contralateral TIA/stroke: NR	Used present on admission designations to determine symptom status at baseline; used ICD-9 codes only for outcome ascertainment; no supplementation with review of medical records; in-hospital outcomes only	Fair
Trials							
Brott, 2010; Silver, 2010	RCT (CREST) 12/2000- 7/2008; asymptomatic patients were only included from 2005 forward	CEA + CAAS CEA: 1,240 (587) CAAS: 1,262 (594)	Multicenter (117 sites)	Asymptomatic patients had to have at least 60% stenosis by angiography, at least 70% by ultrasound, or at least 80% by CT or MR angiography (if the stenosis by ultrasound was initially read as 50%-60%). Asymptomatic defined as symptoms referable only to the hemisphere contralateral to the target vessel or symptoms in either hemisphere >180 days prior to randomization, or vertebrobasilar symptoms only.	CEA/CAAS[e] Mean Age: 70/69 y White: 95%/94% Female: 33%/36% DM: 34%/33% CAD: 44% COPD: NR HF: NR HTN: 88%/88% Smoker: 22%/26% Stenosis: 92%/93% with ≥70% stenosis Prior contralateral CEA: NR Contralateral occlusion: 3%/2% Contralateral TIA/stroke: NR	Unclear whether cases are representative of the source population. A comprehensive training and credentialing process was required of participating interventionalists; only those with low complication rates were invited to participate in the study.	Fair

Table 4. Characteristics of Additional Studies Rated as Good or Fair Quality and Reporting Rates of Periprocedural Complications of CEA or CAAS for Adults With Asymptomatic CAS

Study, Year	Design Study Period	Procedure N Total (N Asymp)	Setting and Source Population	Sample Selection Criteria	Sample Subjects' Characteristics[a]	Threats to Internal and External Validity	Quality
CASANOVA study group, 1991	RCT 1982–1988	CEA: 410 (all) 216 in the group in which all patients had CEA	Patient population recruited from ultrasound labs	Asymptomatic stenosis >50% and <90% Exclusion of MI within past 6 months, renal failure, dementia, severely limited life expectancy	Mean age: 64 White: NR Female: 27% DM: 26% CAD: 44% COPD: NR HF: NR HTN: 59% Smoker: 29% Stenosis: 100% had >50% and <90%; 50% had >70% Prior contralateral CEA: 27% Contralateral occlusion: NR Contralateral TIA/stroke: NR	Subjects from one arm of an RCT; unclear how representative subjects were of overall source population.	Fair
Chaturvedi, 2010 Matsumura, 2010	Uncontrolled trial (CAPTURE-2) 3/2006–1/2009	CAAS: 5,297 (4,337) <80 y: 4,131 (3,388) ≥80 y: 1,177 (949)	CAPTURE-2 is "post-approval" trial to capture rare events	Asymptomatic patients had to have >80% stenosis to have CAAS. Asymptomatic patients had no TIA, amaurosis fugax, or stroke in the territory supplied by the target vessel within 180 days.	Mean Age: 73 y White: NR Female: 39% DM: 37% CAD: 74% COPD: 23% HF: 19% HTN: 89% Smoker: 22% Stenosis: 86% Prior contralateral CEA: 17% Contralateral occlusion: 17% Contralateral TIA/stroke: NR	Unclear whether cases are representative of the source population	Fair
Fairman, 2007	Uncontrolled trial 10/2004–03/2006	CAAS: 3,500 (3,018)	CAPTURE registry: prospective multicenter registry (353 interventionalists) that enrolled high risk surgical patients from 144 sites in US	CAPTURE registry data evaluating stroke rates by various criteria (timing, age, symptom status). Asymptomatic if no TIA, amaurosis fugax, or stroke in the hemisphere supplied by the target vessel within 180 days before procedure.	Mean age: 73 y White: NR Female: 39% DM: 35% CAD: NR COPD: NR HF: 17% HTN: 88% Smoker: 21% Stenosis: mean, 85% Prior contralateral CEA: NR Contralateral occlusion: NR Contralateral TIA/stroke: NR	Unclear whether cases are representative of the source population	Fair

Table 4. Characteristics of Additional Studies Rated as Good or Fair Quality and Reporting Rates of Periprocedural Complications of CEA or CAAS for Adults With Asymptomatic CAS

Study, Year	Design Study Period	Procedure N Total (N Asymp)	Setting and Source Population	Sample Selection Criteria	Sample Subjects' Characteristics[a]	Threats to Internal and External Validity	Quality
Gray, 2009	Pooled analysis of data from 2 uncontrolled trials CAPTURE-2 (3/2006-ongoing as of publication) EXACT (11/2005-4/2007)	CAAS Combined: 6,320 (5,558) EXACT: 2,145 (1,932) Capture-2: 4,175 (3,627)	CAPTURE-2 and EXACT databases; 280 sites and 672 investigators Both are post-marketing registries of CAAS (2 specific devices)	No specific inclusion or exclusion criteria. Asymptomatic patients had no TIA, amaurosis fugax, or stroke in the territory supplied by the target vessel within 180 days.	Combined: Mean Age: 73 y White: NR Female: 38% DM: 36% CAD: 72% COPD: 20% HF: 18% HTN: 90% Smoker: 20% Stenosis: 86% Prior contralateral CEA: NR Contralateral occlusion: 15% Contralateral TIA/stroke: NR	Stroke outcomes assessors were masked, but MI and death were reported by the sites.	Fair
MACE study group, 1992	RCT 1987-1990	CEA: 36 in surgical arm	Mayo Clinic sites (Rochester, Jacksonville, Scottsdale)	Exclusions: age <18 y, women of childbearing age, unstable angina or MI in last 6 months, afib/flutter, severe valvular disease, moderate to severe CHF, severe COPD, cancer, other terminal illness, dementia, other psychiatric illness, renal failure, uncontrolled HTN or DM	Age: 69% >65 y White: 97% Female: 44% DM: 19% CAD: 42% COPD: 0 HF: 0 HTN: 64% Smoker: 25% current; 67% ever Stenosis: NR Prior contralateral CEA: NR Contralateral occlusion: NR Contralateral TIA/stroke: NR	Subjects from one arm of an RCT	Fair
Yadav, 2004	RCT (SAPPHIRE) 8/2000-7/2002	CEA + CAAS: 334 (96) CEA: 167 (46) CAAS: 167 (46)	Multicenter (29 sites)	Symptom status was assessed by a neurologist. Asymptomatic patients were required to have >80% stenosis. All participants had to have one high risk criteria (e.g. severe pulmonary disease, age >80 y).	Mean Age: 73 y White: NR Female: 33% DM: 26% CAD: 81% COPD: 15% HF: 18% HTN: 85% Smoker: 17% Stenosis: NR (inclusion criteria require >80% in asymptomatic patients) Prior contralateral CEA: NR Contralateral occlusion: 24% Contralateral TIA/stroke: NR	Unclear whether cases are representative of the source population. Highly selected surgeons and interventionalists; participating interventionalists had to demonstrate a low complication rate with CEA or CAAS in order to participate in the trial. Unclear whether symptom status was determined using valid and reliable methods.	Fair

Table 4. Characteristics of Additional Studies Rated as Good or Fair Quality and Reporting Rates of Periprocedural Complications of CEA or CAAS for Adults With Asymptomatic CAS

Note: Data are for followup years; reported ages are the mean unless otherwise specified.

[a] Sample characteristics are of entire cohort (symptomatic and asymptomatic patients) unless otherwise noted.
[b] Characteristics are for the asymptomatic subgroup, not whole sample.
[c] Database of abstracted discharge data from national survey of 20% of all nonfederal hospitals in United States; linked to American Hospital Association annual survey of hospitals; asymptomatic if principal discharge diagnosis was CAS "without mention of stroke" with no accompanying secondary diagnoses for TIA.
[d] Arkansas, Georgia, Illinois, Indiana, Iowa, Kentucky, Michigan, Nebraska, Ohio, and Oklahoma.
[e] Patient characteristics are given for asymptomatic patients.
[f] These are for the asymptomatic patient population.

Abbreviations: ACAS = Asymptomatic Carotid Atherosclerosis Study; CAAS = carotid angioplasty and stenting; CABG = coronary artery bypass graft; CAD = coronary artery disease; CAS = carotid artery stenosis; CEA = carotid endarterectomy; CHF = congestive heart failure; COPD = chronic obstructive pulmonary disease; CPT = Current Procedure Terminology; CT = computed tomography; CV = cerebrovascular; DM = diabetes mellitus; HF = heart failure; HMO = health maintenance organization; HTN = hypertension; ICD = International Classification of Diseases; MI = myocardial infarction; MR = magnetic resonance; N = sample size; NIS = Nationwide Inpatient Sample; NR = not reported; RCT = randomized controlled trial; TIA = transient ischemic attack; U/S = ultrasound.

Table 5. Results From Additional Studies Rated as Good or Fair Quality and Reporting Rates of Periprocedural Complications of CEA or CAAS for Adults With Asymptomatic CAS

Study, Year	Method of Outcome Assessment	In-Hospital Rates	30-Day Rates
Cohort studies			
Bratzler, 1996	Standard data collection form; abstractors used administrative data and medical records; also used MedPRO data to identify patients who died or were readmitted with a principal diagnosis of stroke within 30 days.	NR	Combined[a] stroke or death: Overall: 3.7% High[b] volume hospitals: 3.5% Low volume hospitals: 5.2% Stroke: Overall: 2.6% High volume hospitals: 2.8% Low volume hospitals: 1.7% Death: Overall: 1.2% High volume hospitals: 0.7% Low volume hospitals: 3.4%
Cebul, 1998	Administrative data and chart review; trained nurse reviewers to identify outcomes during hospitalization; Medicare Provider Analysis and Review claims to identify all deaths and readmissions within 30 days of CEA, and the records of those were reviewed for occurrence of strokes.	NR	Stroke or death: Overall: 2.4% High volume hospitals: 0% Low volume hospitals: 4.9% Being operated on in a higher volume hospital conferred a 71% reduction in risk for 30-day stroke or death, controlling for indications, comorbid conditions, and surgeon's volume (OR, 0.29 [95% CI, 0.12 to 0.69]). Outcomes did not differ significantly by surgeon volume.
Giacovelli, 2010	ICD-9 codes	Postoperative stroke (Propensity matched): *CEA:* 1.75%; *CAAS:* 2.04% Postoperative TIA (Propensity matched): *CEA:* 0.30%; *CAAS:* 0.32% Postoperative mortality (Propensity matched): *CEA:* 0.39%; *CAAS:* 0.55% Combined postoperative stroke/death (Propensity matched): *CEA:* 1.93%; *CAAS:* 2.37%	NR

Table 5. Results From Additional Studies Rated as Good or Fair Quality and Reporting Rates of Periprocedural Complications of CEA or CAAS for Adults With Asymptomatic CAS

Study, Year	Method of Outcome Assessment	In-Hospital Rates	30-Day Rates
Giles, 2010	ICD-9 codes	Postoperative stroke: *CEA*: 0.6%; *CAAS*: 1.0% Postoperative mortality: *CEA*: 0.4%; *CAAS*: 0.8% Combined postoperative stroke/death: *CEA*: 0.9%; *CAAS*: 1.6%	NR
Halm, 2003; Rockma, 2005; Halm, 2005; Press, 2006	Abstracted from inpatient and outpatient medical records, including all readmissions; 2 investigators independently reviewed records of all those who sustained strokes or TIAs, including 1 neurologist.	NR	Death: 0.57 Nonfatal stroke: 1.69 Death/stroke: 2.26 Nonfatal MI: 0.85
Halm, 2007; Halm, 2009	Medicare claims; ICD-9 codes; hospital records. Research nurses abstracted data from index admission and all readmissions within 30 days of surgery for death, stroke, or TIA. Confirmed by 2 study physicians (including a neurologist). Disagreements resolved by consensus.	NR	Death and stroke: 3.01% Death or stroke in those with high comorbidity: 7.13%[c] Death or stroke rate in those without high comorbidity: 2.69%[c]
Hopkins, 2010 CREST (lead-in/ credentialing)	Stroke severity was judged by a single physician based on chart review.	NR	Death, stroke and MI: 4.8% Death, any stroke: 3.8% Death, major stroke: 1.8% Death: 0.5% Major stroke: 1.6% Minor stroke: 2.0% Age ≤75/ >75 Death, stroke and MI: 3.3%/9.1% Death, any stroke: 2.4%/7.5% Death, major stroke: 1.2%/3.2% Death: 0.5%/0.7% Major stroke: 1.1%/2.9% Minor stroke: 1.2%/4.3%

Table 5. Results From Additional Studies Rated as Good or Fair Quality and Reporting Rates of Periprocedural Complications of CEA or CAAS for Adults With Asymptomatic CAS

Study, Year	Method of Outcome Assessment	In-Hospital Rates	30-Day Rates
Karp, 1998	Claims and medical records. Trained medical abstractors pulled from medical records; a physician reviewed all records in which the abstractor determined that the patient had a stroke to verify and to determine the severity; Deaths from Medicare claims and from Social Security files if the patient died at home.	NR	All strokes:[d] 2.4% Moderate/severe strokes: 1.0% Stroke-related death: 0.2% MI: 0.8% MI-related death: 0.6% Statistically significant increase in morbidity, mortality, and less severe complications at hospitals performing 10 or less CEAs.
Kresowik, 2000	Abstraction from medical records by trained abstractors for index hospitalization and any readmissions; Medicare beneficiary data set to identify deaths within 30 days.	Combined stroke or death: Overall: 2.8% 1994: 2.5% 1995-1996: 2.9%	Combined stroke or death: Overall: 3.4% 1994: 3.8% 1995-1996: 3.3%
Kresowik, 2004	MEDPAR files; ICD-9 codes; Medicare Enrollment Database to identify deaths; comprehensive review of all medical records for the index hospitalization and all admissions within 30 days by trained abstractors.	NR	Combined stroke or death: 1995-1996: 4.1% 1998-1999: 3.8% Death: 1995-1996: 1.1% 1998-1999: 1.0% Combined stroke and death rates (1998-1999) ranged from 1.4% to 6.0% across 10 states; 3 states differed significantly from the mean.
Kresowik, 2001	MEDPAR files; ICD-9 codes; Medicare Enrollment Database to identify deaths; comprehensive review of all medical records for the index hospitalization and all admissions within 30 days by trained abstractors; independent review of strokes by 2 clinicians with expertise in stroke; subset of those classified as having no stroke was also independently reviewed by 2 clinicians.	NR	Combined stroke or death: 3.7%[e] Death: 1.1% Combined stroke and death rates ranged from 2.3% to 6.7% across 10 states; 2 states differed significantly from the mean. Mortality rate ranged from 0.5% to 2.5% across 10 states; 1 state differed significantly from the mean.
McPhee, 2007	ICD-9 codes.	Postoperative stroke: *CEA*: 0.86%; *CAAS*: 1.8% Postoperative mortality: *CEA*: 0.34%; *CAAS*: 0.44% Postoperative MI: *CEA*: 1.7%; *CAAS*: 2.0%	NR

Table 5. Results From Additional Studies Rated as Good or Fair Quality and Reporting Rates of Periprocedural Complications of CEA or CAAS for Adults With Asymptomatic CAS

Study, Year	Method of Outcome Assessment	In-Hospital Rates	30-Day Rates
McPhee, 2008	ICD-9 codes	In-hospital mortality: *CEA*: 0.38%; *CAAS*: 0.57% Postoperative stroke: *CEA*: 0.88%; *CAAS*: 1.6%	NR
Timaran, 2009	ICD-9 codes	Postoperative stroke: *CEA*: 1.0%; *CAAS*: 1.8% In-hospital mortality: *CEA*: 0.5%; *CAAS*: 0.7%	NR
Vouyouka, 2012	ICD-9 codes	Postoperative stroke: *CEA*: 1.54%; *CAAS*: 2.62%; Propensity Matched: *CEA*: 2.05%; *CAAS*: 2.67% Postoperative mortality: *CEA*: 0.33%; *CAAS*: 0.82%; Propensity Matched: *CEA*: 0.39%; *CAAS*: 0.78% Combined postoperative stroke/death: *CEA*: 1.71%; *CAAS*: 3.09%; Propensity Matched: *CEA*: 2.17%; *CAAS*: 3.11%	NR
Young, 2011	ICD-9 codes	In-hospital stroke: *CEA*: 0.88%; *CAAS*: 1.31% In-hospital death: *CEA*: 0.39%; *CAAS*: 0.57% Combined in-hospital stroke/death: *CEA*: 1.16%; *CAAS*: 1.69% In-hospital cardiac complications: *CEA*: 1.86%; *CAAS*: 2.15% Combined in-hospital stroke/death/ cardiac complications: *CEA*: 2.90%; *CAAS*: 3.66%	NR
Yuo, 2013	ICD-9 codes	In-hospital stroke: *CEA*: 1.5%; *CAAS*: 3.2% In-hospital death: *CEA*: 0.5%; *CAAS*: 1.4% Combined in-hospital stroke/death: *CEA*: 1.8%; *CAAS*: 4.1%	NR

Table 5. Results From Additional Studies Rated as Good or Fair Quality and Reporting Rates of Periprocedural Complications of CEA or CAAS for Adults With Asymptomatic CAS

Study, Year Trials	Method of Outcome Assessment	In-Hospital Rates	30-Day Rates
Brott, 2010; Silver, 2010	Neurological exam, including NIHSS assessment and TIA-stroke questionnaire. Study committees unaware of treatment assignment adjudicated stroke and MI events.	NR	CAAS: All patients/patients <80 y MI: 1.2%/0.9% Any stroke: 2.5%/2.4% Major stroke: 0.5%/0.5% Minor stroke: 2.0%/1.8% Any stroke or death: 2.5%/2.4% Any stroke, death or MI: 3.5%/3.1% CEA: MI: 2.2%/2.2% Any stroke: 1.4%/1.5% Major stroke: 0.3%/0.4% Minor stroke: 1.0%/1.1% Any stroke or death: 1.4%/1.5% Any stroke, death or MI: 3.6%/3.7%
CASANOVA study group, 1991	CT scan, neurologic consultant blinded to group assignment.	NR	Death: 1.4% Stroke or death: 3.2% Minor stroke: 0% Lung embolism: 1.4% MI: 0.0% Cranial nerve damage (permanent): 4.2% TIA: 1.9% Cranial nerve damage: 1.4% Pneumonia: 1.4% Local infection: 0% Local hematoma (requiring surgery): 2.8% Other major complication: 1.9% Other minor complication: 0.9%

Table 5. Results From Additional Studies Rated as Good or Fair Quality and Reporting Rates of Periprocedural Complications of CEA or CAAS for Adults With Asymptomatic CAS

Study, Year	Method of Outcome Assessment	In-Hospital Rates	30-Day Rates
Chaturvedi, 2010 Matsumura, 2010	Neurologic assessment at baseline, 24 hours, and 30 days using Health Stroke Scale by an independent neurologist (nonoperator). All strokes and suspected strokes were adjudicated by an independent Clinical Events Adjudication Committee. Death and MI reported by sites.	NR	Death/stroke/MI: 3.0% Death/stroke: 2.8% Death/major stroke: 1.2% Death: 0.7% All stroke: 2.3% Major stroke (all): 0.7% Major ipsilateral stroke: 0.6% Major contralateral stroke: 0.1% Minor stroke (all): 1.6% Minor ipsilateral stroke: 1.4% Minor contralateral stroke: 0.2% MI: 0.3%
Fairman, 2007	Neurologic assessment at baseline, 24 hours, and 30 days using Health Stroke Scale by an independent neurologist (nonoperator). All strokes and suspected strokes were adjudicated by an independent Clinical Events Adjudication Committee (2 independent neurologists). Death and MI reported by sites.	NR	Stroke: 4.1% Major stroke: 1.6%
Gray, 2009	Neurologic assessment at baseline, 24 hours, and 30 days using Health Stroke Scale by an independent neurologist (nonoperator). All strokes and suspected strokes were adjudicated by an independent Clinical Events Adjudication Committee. Death and MI reported by sites.	NR	Full asx sample: Death and stroke: 3.2% Death and major stroke: 1.3% In asx patients age <80 y: Death/stroke: 2.9% Death/major stroke: 1.1% Death: 0.8% Minor stroke: 1.8% Major stroke: 0.6% In asx patients with unfavorable anatomic factors: Death/stroke: 2.7% Death/major stroke: 0.8% Death: 0.3% Minor stroke: 1.9% Major stroke: 0.5%

Table 5. Results From Additional Studies Rated as Good or Fair Quality and Reporting Rates of Periprocedural Complications of CEA or CAAS for Adults With Asymptomatic CAS

Study, Year	Method of Outcome Assessment	In-Hospital Rates	30-Day Rates
MACE study group, 1992	Occurrence and severity of endpoints were adjudicated by 2 participating neurologists and surgeons who were not involved in the management of the patient and who were unaware of the treatment arm; included phone interview 30days after intervention.	NR	TIA: 4% Stroke: 4% MI: 8.3% Minor cranial nerve injury: 11%
Yadav, 2004	Neurological examination, including NIHSS assessment. Major adverse clinical events were adjudicated by an independent, blinded clinical events committee.	NR	CEA: Death, stroke or MI: 10.2% CAAS: Death, stroke or MI: 5.4%

Data are for followup years; reported ages are the mean unless otherwise specified.

[a] The article also reports HTN (3%), wound hematoma (2%), pneumonia (2%), TIA (1%), return to operating room (1%), nerve palsy (1%), acute CHF (<1%), MI (<1%), wound infection (<1%), and other (3%), but the data were not reported separately by symptom status.
[b] High volume = more than 100 Medicare CEAs over the 2 years.
[c] High comorbidity = end stage disease, severe disability, or ≥3 Revised Cardiac Risk Index risk factors.
[d] Article also reports "less serious complications": hematoma (4%) and pneumonia (1.5%), but does not separate by symptom status.
[e] The 1995-1996 data are also included in Kresowik 2004, but results were adjusted for independent clinician validation in Kresowik 2001 (i.e., Kresowik 2004 results were unadjusted, so the numbers are not identical).

Abbreviations: CAAS = carotid angioplasty and stenting; CEA = carotid endarterectomy; CHF = congestive heart failure; COPD = chronic obstructive pulmonary disease; CV = cerebrovascular; HTN = hypertension; ICD = International Classification of Diseases; MI = myocardial infarction; N = sample size; NR = not reported; TIA = transient ischemic attack; U/S = ultrasound.

Table 6. Projected 5-Year Outcomes of Screening 100,000 Asymptomatic Adults for CAS With Duplex Ultrasonography Followed by Confirmatory Testing With MRA

Screening Cascade Component	Variable	CEA	Medical Treatment
Detection	Patients with CAS, n	1,000	1,000
	Positive screening test result (false positive/true positive), n (n/n)	8,860 (7,920/940)	8,860 (7,920/940)
	Patients sent to surgery after MRA confirmation (false positive/true positive), n (n/n)	1,685 (792/893)	NA
Benefits[a]	Any nonperioperative stroke for those with true positive test results, n	53	102
Harms	Perioperative strokes or death, estimated using trial results; using cohort results (false positive/true positive), n (n/n)	41 (19/22); 57 (27/30)	14 (7/7); 2 (1/1)
	Nonfatal perioperative MI, estimated using trial results; using cohort studies (false positive/true positive), n (n/n)	14 (7/7); 14 (7/7)	1 (1/1); 1 (1/1)
	Cranial nerve injuries	64 (30/34)	0 (0/0); 0 (0/0)
	Other complications of surgery: pulmonary embolism, pneumonia, other infection, local hematoma requiring surgery	≤1% estimated each	NA
	Potential psychological harms	Unknown	Unknown
Net for major cardiovascular events avoided or caused[b]	Perioperative stroke/death/MI or any subsequent stroke in patients with either false positive or true positive results: using trial results; using cohort results, n	108; 124	117; 105
	Difference between CEA and medical therapy, using trial results; using cohort results	9 fewer events; 19 more events	10 more events; 19 fewer events
NNS	To prevent 1 major cardiovascular event over about 5 years: using trial results; cohort results	11,111; net harm	NA

Projected benefits and harms were determined for the 1,685 people who would be sent for CEA after MRA confirmation. When relevant, projected outcomes are shown as overall and in parentheses for people who had false positives and those who had true positives to illustrate how many people would undergo unnecessary intervention with resulting harm.

Assumptions were as follows:
1) The true prevalence is 1% in the general asymptomatic primary care population of adults age 65 years and older.
2) Outcomes table based on our findings for CEA; our results suggest that projected outcomes for CAAS are similar or worse; projected outcomes for CAAS were not included in the table.
3) Screening test is carotid duplex ultrasonography, with sensitivity and specificity for CAS of 60% to 99% and 0.94 and 0.92, respectively.
4) Confirmatory test is MRA (sensitivity, 0.95; specificity, 0.90).[47]
5) Rate for any nonperioperative stroke for those with true positive test was based on our meta-analysis, which found a risk difference of -0.055, with rates of 5.9% for the CEA group and 11.4% for the medical therapy group.
6) Perioperative stroke or death rate for CEA is 2.4% when using trial results and 3.3% when using cohort studies of the general population of surgeons and patients.
7) Perioperative stroke or death rate for medical therapy is 0.79% when using trial data and 0.09% when using observational data. We did not estimate zero events for perioperative (i.e., 30-day) stroke or death for the medical therapy group, because some people will have events during that time period.
8) Perioperative nonfatal MI rate for CEA is 0.79% (pooled estimate from ACST and VACS) and 0.056% for medical therapy based on trial results, regardless of whether the test was a true positive or false positive; we estimated a rate of 0.825% for CEA when using cohort studies.[99,103]
9) Cranial nerve injury rate for CEA is 3.8% (as in VACS). The authors reported that functional recovery was observed in all cases and there was no permanent disability. Certainty of this estimate is low as few fair-quality trials or observational studies reported data. One study (CASANOVA) reported higher rates of permanent cranial nerve injury (4.2%).[82] Another study reported a rate of 1.1% for minor cranial nerve injuries.[83]
10) Patients with false positive screening results receive no benefit from either medical therapy or CEA.

[a] Estimates for benefits were based on trial data that have limited applicability to current clinical practice, primarily because medical therapy in trials was ill-defined, varying, and would not have included treatments that are now standard medical therapy. Further, advances in medical therapy have reduced the rate of stroke in people with asymptomatic CAS in recent decades. The true rates for benefit are unknown, and likely less than those reported in trials.
[b] Does not include some important harms from above: cranial nerve injuries, other complications of surgery (pulmonary embolism, pneumonia, other infection, local hematoma requiring surgery), or potential psychological harms.

Abbreviations: CAAS = carotid angioplasty and stenting; CAS = carotid artery stenosis; CEA = carotid endarterectomy; MI = myocardial infarction; MRA = magnetic resonance angiography; NNS = number needed to screen.

Appendix A. Summary of Recommendations for Screening of Asymptomatic CAS Proposed by Expert Panels[a]

Recommendation	Grade/Level of Evidence	Interpretation of Recommendation
American Heart Association/American Stroke Association[21]		
Population screening for asymptomatic carotid stenosis is not recommended.	Class III; Level of Evidence B[b]	Procedure is not effective and may be harmful; evidence from single randomized trial or nonrandomized study
The usefulness of carotid stenting as an alternative to carotid endarterectomy (CEA) in asymptomatic patients at high risk for the surgical procedure is uncertain.	Class IIb; Level of Evidence C	Recommendation's usefulness and efficacy are less established; only diverging expert opinion, case studies, or standard of care
Joint guidelines from multiple U.S. societies (including the American College of Cardiology, American Heart Association, American Stroke Association, American College of Radiology, and the Society for Vascular Surgery)[151]		
It is reasonable to perform duplex ultrasonography to detect hemodynamically significant carotid stenosis in asymptomatic patients with carotid bruit.	Class IIa; Level of Evidence C[b]	Recommendation in favor of treatment or procedure; very limited populations have been evaluated
Duplex ultrasonography to detect hemodynamically significant carotid stenosis may be considered in asymptomatic patients with symptomatic peripheral arterial disease, coronary artery disease, or atherosclerotic aortic aneurysm, but because such patients already have an indication for medical therapy to prevent ischemic symptoms, it is unclear whether establishing the additional diagnosis of extracranial carotid and vertebral artery disease in those without carotid bruit would justify actions that affect clinical outcomes.	Class IIb; Level of Evidence C	Recommendation's usefulness and efficacy is less established; only limited populations have been evaluated
Duplex ultrasonography might be considered to detect carotid stenosis in asymptomatic patients without clinical evidence of atherosclerosis who have ≥2 of the following risk factors: hypertension, hyperlipidemia, tobacco smoking, family history in a 1st-degree relative of atherosclerosis manifested before age 60 years, or family history of ischemic stroke. However, it's unclear whether establishing a diagnosis of extracranial carotid and vertebral artery disease would justify actions that affect clinical outcomes.	Class IIb; Level of Evidence C	Recommendation's usefulness and efficacy are less established; only limited populations have been evaluated
Carotid duplex ultrasonography is not recommended for routine screening of asymptomatic patients who have no clinical manifestations of or risk factors for atherosclerosis.	Class III; Level of Evidence C	Recommendation's usefulness and efficacy are less established; only limited populations have been evaluated
Society for Vascular Surgery Guidelines[152]		
Routine screening is not recommended to detect clinically asymptomatic carotid stenosis in the general population. Screening is not recommended for presence of a neck bruit alone without other risk factors.	Grade I, Level of Evidence A[c]	Risk clearly outweighs benefit, based on high-quality evidence
Screening for asymptomatic clinically significant carotid bifurcation stenosis should be considered in certain groups of patients with multiple risk factors that increase the incidence of disease as long as the patients are fit for and willing to consider carotid intervention if a significant stenosis is discovered. Such groups of patients include those with clinically significant peripheral vascular disease and those age ≥65 years with a history of ≥1 of the following atherosclerotic risk factors: coronary artery disease, smoking, or hypercholesterolemia.	Grade I, Level of Evidence B	Benefit clearly outweighs risk, based on moderate-quality evidence

Appendix A. Summary of Recommendations for Screening of Asymptomatic CAS Proposed by Expert Panels[a]

Recommendation	Grade/Level of Evidence	Interpretation of Recommendation
Carotid screening may be considered in patients prior to coronary artery bypass. Screening is most likely to be fruitful if the patient is age ≥65 years, has left main disease, or has a history of peripheral vascular disease. The strongest indication for screening these patients from the data available is to identify patients at high risk of perioperative stroke.	Grade II, Level of Evidence B	Benefits and risks are more closely matched and more dependent on specific clinical scenarios as well as physician and patient preferences, based on moderate quality evidence

[a] These selected recommendations are most relevant to this review and not meant to be comprehensive. Some recommendations have been summarized.
[b] Recommendations are made using the GRADE (Grades of Recommendation Assessment, Development and Evaluation) system.
[c] Recommendations based on ACCF/AHA Task Force on Practice Guidelines.

Appendix B. Search Strategy

Initial Searches

1/14/13 PubMed

Search	Query	Items found
#1	Search ("Carotid Stenosis"[Mesh] OR "carotid stenosis" OR "carotid artery stenosis")	13181
#2	Search asymptomatic	100045
#3	Search (#1 and #2)	2650
#4	Search "Mass Screening"[Mesh]	92506
#5	Search (#3 and #4)	52
#6	Search "Carotid Stenosis/ultrasonography"[Mesh]	2304
#7	Search "Ultrasonography"[Mesh]	230227
#8	Search (#3 and #7)	590
#9	Search "Endarterectomy, Carotid"[Mesh]	6297
#10	Search (#3 and #9)	1139
#11	Search "Angioplasty"[Mesh]	51935
#12	Search (#3 and #11)	451
#13	Search "Magnetic Resonance Angiography"[Mesh]	15076
#14	Search (#3 and #13)	86
#15	Search ("Angioplasty, Balloon"[Mesh] OR "balloon dilation")	47673
#16	Search (#3 and #15)	228
#17	Search "Stents"[Mesh]	47106
#18	Search (#3 and #17)	602
#19	Search ("CT angiography"[tiab] OR "computed tomographic angiography"[tiab])	6410
#20	Search (#3 and #19)	32
#21	Search "Carotid Stenosis/radiography"[Mesh]	1613
#22	Search (#3 and #21)	236
#23	Search (#5 or #6 or #8 or #10 or #12 or #14 or #16 or #18 or #20 or #22)	3798
#24	Search ("Randomized Controlled Trial"[Publication Type] OR "Single-Blind Method"[MeSH] OR "Double-Blind Method"[MeSH] OR "Random Allocation"[MeSH] OR trial[tiab])	615495
#25	Search (#23 and #24)	448
#26	Search (("review"[Publication Type] AND "systematic"[tiab]) OR "systematic review"[All Fields] OR ("review literature as topic"[MeSH] AND "systematic"[tiab]) OR "meta-analysis"[Publication Type] OR "meta-analysis as topic"[MeSH Terms] OR "meta-analysis"[All Fields])	101498
#27	Search (#23 and #26)	68
#28	Search (#25 or #27)	498
#29	Search ("stroke"[MeSH Terms] OR "stroke"[All Fields] OR "brain infarction"[All Fields] OR "cerebrovascular disorder"[All Fields] OR "cerebrovascular disease"[All Fields] OR "CVA"[All Fields] OR "cerebral infarction"[All Fields] OR "ischemic stroke"[All Fields] OR (("stroke"[MeSH Terms] OR "stroke"[All Fields]) AND ("ischemia"[MeSH Terms] OR "ischemia"[All Fields] OR "ischemic"[All Fields])) OR "cerebrovascular accident"[All Fields])	201437
#30	Search ("risk"[MeSH Terms] OR "risk assessment"[MeSH Terms] OR "risk adjustment"[MeSH Terms] OR "risk assessment"[MeSH Terms] OR ("risk"[All Fields] AND "assessment"[All Fields]) OR "risk assessment"[All Fields] OR ("assessment"[All Fields] AND "benefit"[All Fields] AND "risk"[All Fields]) OR ("assessments"[All Fields] AND "benefit"[All Fields] AND "risk"[All Fields]))	799562
#31	Search (#3 and #29 and #30)	818
#32	Search (#31 and #24)	132
#33	Search ("Case-Control Studies"[MeSH] OR "Cohort Studies"[MeSH] OR "comparative study"[pt] OR "Epidemiologic Studies"[MeSH] OR "Cross-Over Studies"[MeSH] OR "Follow-Up Studies"[MeSH] OR "observational study" OR "observational studies" OR "cohort"[tw] OR "case control"[tw])	2911595
#34	Search (#31 and #33)	484
#35	Search (#32 or #34)	524
#36	Search (#5 or #6 or #8 or #14 or #20 or #22)	2774
#37	Search (#36 and #26)	29
#38	Search ("Endarterectomy, Carotid/statistics and numerical data"[Mesh])	769

Search	Query	Items found
#39	Search "Endarterectomy, Carotid/adverse effects"[Mesh]	1573
#40	Search (#23 or #38 or #39)	5322
#41	Search (harm OR harms OR adverse effect* OR adverse event* OR complication* OR death OR stroke OR "Myocardial Infarction"[Mesh] OR "myocardial infarction" OR (unnecessary AND "carotid endarterectomy") OR "Kidney Failure, Chronic"[Mesh] OR "Renal Insufficiency"[Mesh] OR "Cranial Nerve Diseases"[Mesh] OR "Cranial Nerve Injuries"[Mesh] OR (neck AND hematoma*))	3944352
#42	Search (#40 and #41)	4080
#43	Search (comment[pt] OR editorial[pt] OR letter[pt] OR news[pt])	1348329
#44	Search (#25 or #27) Filters: Humans	494
#45	Search (#25 or #27) Filters: Humans; English	458
#46	Search (#25 or #27) Filters: Humans; English; Adult: 19+ years	283
#47	Search (#46 NOT #43)	283
#48	Search (#32 or #34) Filters: Humans	524
#49	Search (#32 or #34) Filters: Humans; English	485
#50	Search (#32 or #34) Filters: Humans; English; Adult: 19+ years	414
#51	Search (#50 NOT #43)	413
#52	Search (#36 and #26) Filters: Humans	28
#53	Search (#36 and #26) Filters: Humans; English	26
#54	Search (#36 and #26) Filters: Humans; English; Adult: 19+ years	7
#55	Search (#54 NOT #43)	7
#56	Search (#40 and #41) Filters: Humans	4056
#57	Search (#40 and #41) Filters: Humans; English	3666
#58	Search (#40 and #41) Filters: Humans; English; Adult: 19+ years	2606
#59	Search (#58 NOT #43)	2548
#60	Search (#47 or #51 or #55 or #59)	2667

1/14/13 Cochrane Library

ID	Search	Hits
#1	[mh "Carotid Stenosis"] or "carotid stenosis" or "carotid artery stenosis"	817
#2	asymptomatic	5592
#3	#1 and #2	254
#4	[mh "Mass Screening"]	4250
#5	#3 and #4	7
#6	[mh "Carotid Stenosis"/US]	109
#7	[mh Ultrasonography]	6706
#8	#3 and #7	47
#9	[mh "Endarterectomy, Carotid"]	442
#10	#3 and #9	121
#11	[mh Angioplasty]	3950
#12	#3 and #11	36
#13	[mh "Magnetic Resonance Angiography"]	338
#14	#3 and #13	4
#15	[mh "Angioplasty, Balloon"] or "balloon dilation"	4135
#16	#3 and #15	19
#17	[mh Stents]	2939
#18	#3 and #17	49
#19	"CT angiography" or "computed tomographic angiography"	242
#20	#3 and #19	3
#21	[mh "Carotid Stenosis"/RA]	52
#22	#3 and #21	11
#23	#5 or #6 or #8 or #10 or #12 or #14 or #16 or #18 or #20 or #22	242
#24	"Randomized Controlled Trial" or rct or "Single-Blind Method" or "Double-Blind Method" or "Random Allocation" or trial	716586

Appendix B. Search Strategy

ID	Search	Hits
#25	#23 and #24	220
#26	(review and systematic) or "systematic review" or ([mh "review literature as topic"] and systematic) or "meta-analysis" or [mh "meta-analysis as topic"]	36928
#27	#23 and #26	47
#28	#25 or #27	226
#29	[mh stroke] or stroke or "brain infarction" or "cerebrovascular disorder" or "cerebrovascular disease" or CVA or "cerebral infarction" or "ischemic stroke" or (stroke and (ischemia or ischemic)) or "cerebrovascular accident"	28247
#30	[mh risk] or [mh "risk assessment"] or [mh "risk adjustment"] or (risk and assessment) or "risk assessment"	46693
#31	#3 and #29 and #30	111
#32	#31 and #24	99
#33	"Case-Control Studies" or "Cohort Studies" or "comparative study" or "Epidemiologic Studies" or "Cross-Over Studies" or "Follow-Up Studies" or "observational study" or "observational studies" or "cohort" or "case control"	200532
#34	#31 and #33	57
#35	#32 or #34	104
#36	#5 or #6 or #8 or #14 or #20 or #22	141
#37	#36 and #26	12
#38	[mh "Endarterectomy, Carotid"/SN]	15
#39	[mh "Endarterectomy, Carotid"/AE]	110
#40	#23 or #38 or #39	322
#41	harm or harms or adverse effect* or adverse event* or complication* or death or stroke or [mh "Myocardial Infarction"] or "myocardial infarction" or (unnecessary and "carotid endarterectomy") or [mh "Kidney Failure, Chronic"] or [mh "Renal Insufficiency"] or [mh "Cranial Nerve Diseases"] or [mh "Cranial Nerve Injuries"] or (neck and hematoma*)	229088
#42	#40 and #41	295
#43	comment:pt or editorial:pt or letter:pt or news:pt	6335
#44	#28 not #43	223
#45	#35 not #43	104
#46	#37 not #43	12
#47	#42 not #43	293
#48	#44 or #45 or #46 or #47	330

1/14/13 Embase

Search	Query	Items Found
#52	#45 OR #47 OR #49 OR #51 AND [embase]/lim	1,805
#51	#50 NOT #43 AND [embase]/lim	1,618
#50	#42 AND ([adult]/lim OR [aged]/lim) AND [humans]/lim AND [english]/lim AND [embase]/lim	1,652
#49	#48 NOT #43 AND [embase]/lim	45
#48	#37 AND ([adult]/lim OR [aged]/lim) AND [humans]/lim AND [english]/lim AND [embase]/lim	45
#47	#46 NOT #43 AND [embase]/lim	252
#46	#35 AND ([adult]/lim OR [aged]/lim) AND [humans]/lim AND [english]/lim AND [embase]/lim	254
#45	#44 NOT #43 AND [embase]/lim	430
#44	#28 AND ([adult]/lim OR [aged]/lim) AND [humans]/lim AND [english]/lim AND [embase]/lim	432
#43	'editorial'/exp OR 'letter'/exp AND [embase]/lim	902,998
#42	#40 AND #41 AND [embase]/lim	3,297
#41	Harm OR harms OR adverse AND effect* OR 'adverse outcome'/exp OR 'adverse event' OR 'adverse events' OR complication* OR 'death'/exp OR 'stroke'/exp OR 'heart infarction'/exp OR 'myocardial infarction'/exp OR (unnecessary AND 'carotid endarterectomy'/exp) OR 'chronic kidney failure'/exp OR 'kidney failure'/exp OR 'cranial neuropathy'/exp OR 'cranial nerve injury'/exp OR ('neck'/exp AND hematoma*) AND [embase]/lim	2,755,904
#40	#23 OR #38 OR #39 AND [embase]/lim	5,265
#39	'carotid endarterectomy'/exp AND 'adverse outcome'/exp AND [embase]/lim	33
#38	'carotid endarterectomy'/exp AND 'health statistics'/exp AND [embase]/lim	2

Appendix B. Search Strategy

Search	Query	Items Found
#37	#36 AND #26 AND [embase]/lim	420
#36	#5 OR OR #6 OR #8 OR #14 OR #20 OR #22 AND [embase]/lim	3,859
#35	#32 OR #34 AND [embase]/lim	650
#34	#31 AND #33 AND [embase]/lim	433
#33	'cohort analysis'/exp OR 'comparative study'/exp OR 'epidemiological study' OR 'crossover procedure'/exp OR 'follow up'/exp OR 'case control study'/exp OR 'observational study'/exp OR 'observational studies'/exp OR cohort AND [embase]/lim	1,315,793
#32	#31 AND #24 AND [embase]/lim	371
#31	#3 AND #29 AND #30 AND [embase]/lim	1,290
#30	'risk'/exp OR 'risk assessment'/exp OR 'risk adjustment'/exp OR ('risk'/exp AND assessment) OR (assessment AND benefit AND 'risk'/exp) OR (assessments AND benefit AND 'risk'/exp) AND [embase]/lim	1,043,208
#29	'stroke'/exp OR 'brain infarction'/exp OR 'cerebrovascular disease'/exp OR 'cerebral infarction'/exp OR 'brain ischemia'/exp OR ischemic OR 'ischemia'/exp OR 'cerebrovascular accident'/exp OR 'cva'/exp AND [embase]/lim	742,015
#28	#25 OR #27 AND [embase]/lim	1,385
#27	#23 AND #26 AND [embase]/lim	671
#26	'review'/ exp OR (systematic AND 'review'/exp) OR 'systematic review'/exp OR ('literature'/exp AND 'review'/exp AND systematic) OR 'meta analysis (topic)'/exp OR 'meta analysis'/exp AND [embase]/lim	1,328,033
#25	#23 AND #24 AND [embase]/lim	987
#24	'randomized controlled trial'/exp OR 'single blind procedure'/exp OR 'double blind procedure'/exp OR 'random allocation'/exp OR trial AND [embase]/lim	1,012,147
#23	#5 OR #6 OR #8 OR #10 OR #12 OR #14 OR #16 OR #18 OR #20 OR #22 AND [embase]/lim	5,239
#22	#3 AND #21 AND [embase]/lim	3
#21	'carotid artery obstruction'/exp/dm_rt AND [embase]/lim	11
#20	#3 AND #19 AND [embase]/lim	94
#19	'computed tomographic angiography'/exp AND [embase]/lim	17,301
#18	#3 AND #17 AND [embase]/lim	626
#17	'stent'/exp AND [embase]/lim	76,186
#16	#3 AND #15 AND [embase]/lim	74
#15	'carotid angioplasty'/exp OR 'balloon dilatation'/exp AND [embase]/lim	8,331
#14	#3 AND #13 AND [embase]/lim	159
#13	'magnetic resonance angiography'/exp AND [embase]/lim	18,209
#12	#3 AND #11 AND [embase]/lim	707
#11	'angioplasty'/exp AND [embase]/lim	50,229
#10	#3 AND #9 AND [embase]/lim	1,414
#9	'carotid endarterectomy'/exp AND [embase]/lim	10,608
#8	#3 AND #7	727
#7	'echography'/exp AND [embase]/lim	376,374
#6	'carotid artery obstruction'/exp AND 'echography'/exp AND [embase]/lim	3,724
#5	#3 AND #4 AND [embase]/lim	10
#4	'mass screening'/exp AND [embase]/lim	100,488
#3	#1 AND #2 AND [embase]/lim	2,998
#2	asymptomatic AND [embase]/lim	106,122
#1	'carotid artery obstruction'/exp OR 'carotid stenosis'/exp OR 'carotid artery stenosis'/exp AND [embase]/lim	19,804

Additional searches (for drugs) for KQ 6 (PubMed and Cochrane Library)

4/11/13 PubMed

Search	Query	Items found
#19	Search "Carotid Stenosis"[Mesh] OR "carotid stenosis" OR "carotid artery stenosis"	13363
#20	Search asymptomatic	101659
#21	Search (#19 and #20)	2691

Appendix B. Search Strategy

#22	Search ("Aspirin"[Mesh] OR "Hydroxymethylglutaryl-CoA Reductase Inhibitors" [Pharmacological Action] OR statins[tiab] OR "Platelet Aggregation Inhibitors"[Mesh] OR "Drug Therapy"[Mesh] OR "drug therapy"[subheading])	2173853
#23	Search (#21 and #22)	240
#29	Search ("Chemicals and Drugs Category"[Mesh])	10950565
#30	Search (#21 and #29)	508
#31	Search (#30 NOT #23)	318
#32	Search ("Randomized Controlled Trial"[Publication Type] OR "Single-Blind Method"[MeSH] OR "Double-Blind Method"[MeSH] OR "Random Allocation"[MeSH] OR trial[tiab])	625507
#33	Search (#31 and #32)	18
#34	Search (#31 and #32) Filters: Humans	18
#35	Search (#31 and #32) Filters: Humans; English	15
#36	Search (#31 and #32) Filters: Humans; English; Adult: 19+ years	13
#37	Search (("review"[Publication Type] AND "systematic"[tiab]) OR "systematic review"[All Fields] OR ("review literature as topic"[MeSH] AND "systematic"[tiab]) OR "meta-analysis"[Publication Type] OR "meta-analysis as topic"[MeSH Terms] OR "meta-analysis"[All Fields]) Filters: Humans; English; Adult: 19+ years	19048
#38	Search (#31 and #37) Filters: Humans; English; Adult: 19+ years	0
#39	Search (Chlorthalidone[mesh] AND #31)	0
#40	Search (Chlorthalidone[mesh] and #21)	0
#42	Search (Hydrochlorothiazide[mesh] AND #21)	3
#43	Search (#42 and (#32 or #37)) Filters: Humans; English; Adult: 19+ years	3
#44	Search (#43 NOT (#23 or #36)) Filters: Humans; English; Adult: 19+ years	0
#45	Search ("Lisinopril"[Mesh] AND #21) Filters: Humans; English; Adult: 19+ years	0
#46	Search ("Atenolol"[Mesh] AND #21) Filters: Humans; English; Adult: 19+ years	0
#47	Search (Metoprolol[Mesh] AND #21) Filters: Humans; English; Adult: 19+ years	0

4/11/13 Cochrane Library (3 results; 1 Cochrane review and 2 trials. All 3 were retrieved in previous searches.)

ID	Search	Hits
#1	[mh "Carotid Stenosis"] or "carotid stenosis" or "carotid artery stenosis"	827
#2	asymptomatic	5655
#3	#1 and #2	260
#4	[mh Aspirin] or [mh "Hydroxymethylglutaryl-CoA Reductase Inhibitors"] or (statins:ti or statins:ab) or [mh "Platelet Aggregation Inhibitors"] or [mh "Drug Therapy"] or [mh /DT]	200682
#5	#3 and #4	35
#6	[mh "Pharmacologic Actions"]	156873
#7	#3 and #6	23
#8	#7 not #5	3

CAS Gray Literature Searches

A) WHO ICTRP (*International Clinical Trials Registry Platform*) search 2-12-13
   1. 16 results for Title search: "carotid stenosis" OR "carotid artery stenosis"

   2. 32 results for Condition search: "carotid stenosis" OR "carotid artery stenosis"

B) ClinicalTrials.gov search 2-12-13 (94 trials)
(("carotid stenosis" OR "carotid artery stenosis" AND asymptomatic) AND ("Mass Screening" OR screening OR Ultrasonography OR "carotid endarterectomy" OR Angioplasty OR "Magnetic Resonance Angiography" OR "balloon angioplasty" OR "balloon dilation" OR stent* OR "CT angiography" OR "computed tomographic angiography" OR radiography)) [ALL-FIELDS]

C) We said we would search Cochrane Stroke Group Trials registry, but I could not figure out how to search for *trials* specifically within that group, so I repeated a search in Cochrane Central Register of Controlled Trials (CENTRAL) limited to trials and groups, but did not limit to study types except to remove editorials, letter, comments, news; and found **170** results. I checked this against our original Cochrane search and it should add 120 new citations and discard 50 duplicates. Here is the search:

2/11/13 Cochrane Trials Search

ID	Search	Hits
#1	[mh "carotid stenosis"] or "carotid stenosis" or "carotid artery stenosis"	822
#2	asymptomatic	5618
#3	#1 and #2	258
#4	[mh "mass screening"]	4337
#5	#3 and #4	7
#6	[mh "carotid stenosis"/US]	109
#7	[mh ultrasonography]	6749
#8	#3 and #7	47
#9	[mh "endarterectomy, carotid"]	446
#10	#3 and #9	124
#11	[mh angioplasty]	3972
#12	#3 and #11	38
#13	[mh "Magnetic Resonance Angiography"]	340
#14	#3 and #13	4
#15	[mh "angioplasty, balloon"] or "balloon dilation"	4150
#16	#3 and #15	19
#17	[mh stents]	2971
#18	#3 and #17	51
#19	"CT angiography":ti or "CT angiography":ab or "computed tomographic angiography":ti or "computed tomographic angiography":ab	186
#20	#3 and #19	2
#21	[mh "carotid stenosis"/RA]	52
#22	#3 and #21	11
#23	#5 or #6 or #8 or #10 or #12 or #14 or #16 or #18 or #20 or #22	244
#24	comment:pt or editoral:pt or letter:pt or news:pt	6182
#25	#23 not #24 in Trials and Cochrane Groups	170

Bridge Searches

9/27/13 and 10/3/13

Search	Query	Items found
#1	Search ("Carotid Stenosis"[Mesh] OR "carotid stenosis" OR "carotid artery stenosis")	13743
#2	Search asymptomatic	104694
#3	Search (#1 and #2)	2770
#4	Search "Aspirin"[Mesh]	36926
#5	Search (#3 and #4)	73
#6	Search "Hydroxymethylglutaryl-CoA Reductase Inhibitors"[Mesh]	18957
#7	Search "Hydroxymethylglutaryl-CoA Reductase Inhibitors" [Pharmacological Action]	27130
#8	Search (#6 or #7)	27130
#9	Search (#3 and #8)	39
#10	Search (#3 AND statins[tiab])	39
#11	Search (#9 or #10)	63
#12	Search "Platelet Aggregation Inhibitors"[Mesh]	25236
#13	Search (#3 and #12)	79
#14	Search "Drug Therapy"[Mesh]	1006539
#15	Search "drug therapy"[subheading]	1621742
#16	Search (#14 or #15)	2176937
#17	Search (#3 and #16)	159
#18	Search (#5 or #11 or #13 or #17)	251
#19	Search ("Randomized Controlled Trial"[Publication Type] OR "Single-Blind Method"[MeSH] OR	645662

Appendix B. Search Strategy

"Double-Blind Method"[MeSH] OR "Random Allocation"[MeSH] OR trial[tiab])

#20	Search (#18 and #19)	69
#21	Search (("review"[Publication Type] AND "systematic"[tiab]) OR "systematic review"[All Fields] OR ("review literature as topic"[MeSH] AND "systematic"[tiab]) OR "meta-analysis"[Publication Type] OR "meta-analysis as topic"[MeSH Terms] OR "meta-analysis"[All Fields])	114200
#22	Search (#18 and #21)	13
#23	Search (#20 or #22)	79
#24	Search (#20 or #22) Filters: Humans	76
#25	Search (#20 or #22) Filters: Humans; English	72
#26	Search (#20 or #22) Filters: Humans; English; Adult: 19+ years	44
#27	Search ("retraction"[All Fields] OR "Retracted Publication"[pt] AND #18)	0
#28	Search (#20 or #22) Filters: Publication date from 2013/01/01 to 2013/12/31; Humans; English; Adult: 19+ years	2

03/10/13 Cochrane Update Search for Statins (4 New)

ID	Search	Hits
#1	[mh "Carotid Stenosis"] or "carotid stenosis" or "carotid artery stenosis"	853
#2	asymptomatic	5775
#3	#1 and #2	268
#4	[mh Aspirin]	657
#5	#3 and #4	4
#6	[mh "Hydroxymethylglutaryl-CoA Reductase Inhibitors"]	2444
#7	#3 and #6	2
#8	#3 and (statins:ti or statins:ab)	2
#9	[mh "Platelet Aggregation Inhibitors"]	2762
#10	#3 and #9	12
#11	[mh "Drug Therapy"] or [mh /DT]	202679
#12	#3 and #11	32
#13	#5 or #7 or #8 or #10 or #12 from 2012 to 2013	4

9/27/13 PubMed (63 results) and Retractions (3) (KQs 1-5, 7, and 8 search [separate/additional searches were conducted for KQ 6])

Search	Query	Items found
#1	Search "Carotid Stenosis"[Mesh] OR "carotid stenosis" OR "carotid artery stenosis"	13732
#2	Search asymptomatic	104580
#3	Search (#1 and #2)	2768
#4	Search "Mass Screening"[Mesh]	95673
#5	Search (#3 and #4)	53
#6	Search "Carotid Stenosis/ultrasonography"[Mesh]	2371
#7	Search "Ultrasonography"[Mesh]	238537
#8	Search (#3 and #7)	619
#9	Search "Endarterectomy, Carotid"[Mesh]	6520
#10	Search (#3 and #9)	1188
#11	Search "Angioplasty"[Mesh]	53078
#12	Search (#3 and #11)	469
#13	Search "Magnetic Resonance Angiography"[Mesh]	15908
#14	Search (#3 and #13)	90
#15	Search ("Angioplasty, Balloon"[Mesh] OR "balloon dilation")	48723
#16	Search (#3 and #15)	235
#17	Search "Stents"[Mesh]	49701
#18	Search (#3 and #17)	640
#19	Search ("CT angiography"[tiab] OR "computed tomographic angiography"[tiab])	7038
#20	Search (#3 and #19)	36
#21	Search "Carotid Stenosis/radiography"[Mesh]	1664
#22	Search (#3 and #21)	246
#23	Search (#5 or #6 or #8 or #10 or #12 or #14 or #16 or #18 or #20 or #22)	3937
#24	Search ("Randomized Controlled Trial"[Publication Type] OR "Single-Blind Method"[MeSH] OR	645006

Appendix B. Search Strategy

Search	Query	Items found
	"Double-Blind Method"[MeSH] OR "Random Allocation"[MeSH] OR trial[tiab])	
#25	Search (#23 and #24)	462
#26	Search (("review"[Publication Type] AND "systematic"[tiab]) OR "systematic review"[All Fields] OR ("review literature as topic"[MeSH] AND "systematic"[tiab]) OR "meta-analysis"[Publication Type] OR "meta-analysis as topic"[MeSH Terms] OR "meta-analysis"[All Fields])	113879
#27	Search (#23 and #26)	75
#28	Search (#25 or #27)	518
#29	Search ("stroke"[MeSH Terms] OR "stroke"[All Fields] OR "brain infarction"[All Fields] OR "cerebrovascular disorder"[All Fields] OR "cerebrovascular disease"[All Fields] OR "CVA"[All Fields] OR "cerebral infarction"[All Fields] OR "ischemic stroke"[All Fields] OR (("stroke"[MeSH Terms] OR "stroke"[All Fields]) AND ("ischemia"[MeSH Terms] OR "ischemia"[All Fields] OR "ischemic"[All Fields])) OR "cerebrovascular accident"[All Fields])	213772
#30	Search ("risk"[MeSH Terms] OR "risk assessment"[MeSH Terms] OR "risk adjustment"[MeSH Terms] OR "risk assessment"[MeSH Terms] OR ("risk"[All Fields] AND "assessment"[All Fields]) OR "risk assessment"[All Fields] OR ("assessment"[All Fields] AND "benefit"[All Fields] AND "risk"[All Fields]) OR ("assessments"[All Fields] AND "benefit"[All Fields] AND "risk"[All Fields]))	843578
#31	Search (#3 and #29 and #30)	861
#32	Search (#31 and #24)	138
#33	Search ("Case-Control Studies"[MeSH] OR "Cohort Studies"[MeSH] OR "comparative study"[pt] OR "Epidemiologic Studies"[MeSH] OR "Cross-Over Studies"[MeSH] OR "Follow-Up Studies"[MeSH] OR "observational study" OR "observational studies" OR "cohort"[tw] OR "case control"[tw])	3019090
#34	Search (#31 and #33)	508
#35	Search (#32 or #34)	551
#36	Search (#5 or #6 or #8 or #14 or #20 or #22)	2868
#37	Search (#36 and #26)	29
#38	Search ("Endarterectomy, Carotid/statistics and numerical data"[Mesh])	813
#39	Search "Endarterectomy, Carotid/adverse effects"[Mesh]	1666
#40	Search (#23 or #38 or #39)	5541
#41	Search (harm OR harms OR adverse effect* OR adverse event* OR complication* OR death OR stroke OR "Myocardial Infarction"[Mesh] OR "myocardial infarction" OR (unnecessary AND "carotid endarterectomy") OR "Kidney Failure, Chronic"[Mesh] OR "Renal Insufficiency"[Mesh] OR "Cranial Nerve Diseases"[Mesh] OR "Cranial Nerve Injuries"[Mesh] OR (neck AND hematoma*))	4084165
#42	Search (#40 and #41)	4269
#43	Search (comment[pt] OR editorial[pt] OR letter[pt] OR news[pt])	1407811
#44	Search (#25 or #27) Filters: Humans	515
#45	Search (#25 or #27) Filters: Humans; English	478
#46	Search (#25 or #27) Filters: Humans; English; Adult: 19+ years	293
#47	Search (#46 NOT #43)	293
#48	Search (#32 or #34) Filters: Humans	551
#49	Search (#32 or #34) Filters: Humans; English	512
#50	Search (#32 or #34) Filters: Humans; English; Adult: 19+ years	439
#51	Search (#50 NOT #43)	438
#52	Search (#36 and #26) Filters: Humans	29
#53	Search (#36 and #26) Filters: Humans; English	27
#54	Search (#36 and #26) Filters: Humans; English; Adult: 19+ years	7
#55	Search (#54 NOT #43)	7
#56	Search (#40 and #41) Filters: Humans	4245
#57	Search (#40 and #41) Filters: Humans; English	3832
#58	Search (#40 and #41) Filters: Humans; English; Adult: 19+ years	2732
#59	Search (#58 NOT #43)	2673
#60	Search (#47 or #51 or #55 or #59)	2795
#61	Search (#60 AND (2012/12/14:2013/09/27[edat]))	**63**
#62	Search (#21 or #31 or #42)	5732
#63	Search (#62 AND ("retraction"[All Fields] OR "Retracted Publication"[pt]))	**3**

Appendix B. Search Strategy

KQ 6 Search Update for Additional Drugs (1 new RCT and 0 retractions. The 1 new RCT was a duplicate with the search above and was discarded.)

Search	Query	Items found
#1	Search ("Carotid Stenosis"[Mesh] OR "carotid stenosis" OR "carotid artery stenosis")	13732
#2	Search asymptomatic	104580
#3	Search (#1 and #2)	2768
#4	Search ("Aspirin"[Mesh] OR "Hydroxymethylglutaryl-CoA Reductase Inhibitors" [Pharmacological Action] OR statins[tiab] OR "Platelet Aggregation Inhibitors"[Mesh] OR "Drug Therapy"[Mesh] OR "drug therapy"[subheading])	2222027
#5	Search (#3 and #4)	251
#6	Search ("Chemicals and Drugs Category"[Mesh])	11152919
#7	Search (#3 and #6)	533
#8	Search (#7 NOT #5)	332
#9	Search ("Randomized Controlled Trial"[Publication Type] OR "Single-Blind Method"[MeSH] OR "Double-Blind Method"[MeSH] OR "Random Allocation"[MeSH] OR trial[tiab])	645006
#10	Search (#8 and #9)	19
#11	Search (#8 and #9) Filters: Humans	19
#12	Search (#8 and #9) Filters: Humans; English	16
#13	Search (#8 and #9) Filters: Humans; English; Adult: 19+ years	14
#14	Search (("review"[Publication Type] AND "systematic"[tiab]) OR "systematic review"[All Fields] OR ("review literature as topic"[MeSH] AND "systematic"[tiab]) OR "meta-analysis"[Publication Type] OR "meta-analysis as topic"[MeSH Terms] OR "meta-analysis"[All Fields])) Filters: Humans; English; Adult: 19+ years	20306
#15	Search (#8 and #14) Filters: Humans; English; Adult: 19+ years	0
#16	Search (Chlorthalidone[mesh] AND #8)	0
#17	Search (Chlorthalidone[mesh] AND #3)	0
#18	Search (Hydrochlorothiazide[mesh] AND #3)	3
#19	Search (#18 AND (#9 or #14))	3
#20	Search (#18 AND (#9 or #14)) Filters: Humans	3
#21	Search (#18 AND (#9 or #14)) Filters: Humans; English	3
#22	Search (#18 AND (#9 or #14)) Filters: Humans; English; Adult: 19+ years	3
#23	Search (#22 NOT (#5 or #13)) Filters: Humans; English; Adult: 19+ years	0
#24	Search ("Lisinopril"[Mesh] AND #3) Filters: Humans; English; Adult: 19+ years	0
#25	Search ("Atenolol"[Mesh] AND #3) Filters: Humans; English; Adult: 19+ years	0
#26	Search ("Metoprolol"[Mesh] AND #3) Filters: Humans; English; Adult: 19+ years	0
#27	Search (#13 AND (2013/03/11:2013/09/27[edat])) Filters: Humans; English; Adult: 19+ years	1

9/27/2013 Cochrane Library Update Search

ID	Search	Hits
#1	[mh "Carotid Stenosis"] or "carotid stenosis" or "carotid artery stenosis"	853
#2	asymptomatic	5772
#3	#1 and #2	268
#4	[mh "Mass Screening"]	4548
#5	#3 and #4	7
#6	[mh "Carotid Stenosis"/US]	112
#7	[mh Ultrasonography]	6996
#8	#3 and #7	48
#9	[mh "Endarterectomy, Carotid"]	461
#10	#3 and #9	129
#11	[mh Angioplasty]	4239
#12	#3 and #11	38
#13	[mh "Magnetic Resonance Angiography"]	350
#14	#3 and #13	5
#15	[mh "Angioplasty, Balloon"] or "balloon dilation"	4026
#16	#3 and #15	19
#17	[mh Stents]	3110
#18	#3 and #17	54
#19	"CT angiography" or "computed tomographic angiography"	275

Appendix B. Search Strategy

ID	Search	Hits
#20	#3 and #19	3
#21	[mh "Carotid Stenosis"/RA]	53
#22	#3 and #21	11
#23	[mh Aspirin] or [mh "Hydroxymethylglutaryl-CoA Reductase Inhibitors"] or (statins:ti or statins:ab) or [mh "Platelet Aggregation Inhibitors"] or [mh "Drug Therapy"] or [mh /DT]	204690
#24	#3 and #23	38
#25	[mh "Pharmacologic Actions"]	160591
#26	#3 and #25	25
#27	#26 not #24	3
#28	#5 or #6 or #8 or #10 or #12 or #14 or #16 or #18 or #20 or #22 or #27	255
#29	"Randomized Controlled Trial" or rct or "Single-Blind Method" or "Double-Blind Method" or "Random Allocation" or trial	750415
#30	#28 and #29	230
#31	(review and systematic) or "systematic review" or ([mh "review literature as topic"] and systematic) or "meta-analysis" or [mh "meta-analysis as topic"]	43560
#32	#28 and #31	51
#33	#30 or #32	236
#34	[mh stroke] or stroke or "brain infarction" or "cerebrovascular disorder" or "cerebrovascular disease" or CVA or "cerebral infarction" or "ischemic stroke" or (stroke and (ischemia or ischemic)) or "cerebrovascular accident"	29927
#35	[mh risk] or [mh "risk assessment"] or [mh "risk adjustment"] or (risk and assessment) or "risk assessment"	50215
#36	#3 and #34 and #35	117
#37	#36 and #29	104
#38	"Case-Control Studies" or "Cohort Studies" or "comparative study" or "Epidemiologic Studies" or "Cross-Over Studies" or "Follow-Up Studies" or "observational study" or "observational studies" or "cohort" or "case control"	206465
#39	#36 and #38	61
#40	#37 or #39	109
#41	#5 or #6 or #8 or #14 or #20 or #22	146
#42	#41 and #31	12
#43	[mh "Endarterectomy, Carotid"/SN]	16
#44	[mh "Endarterectomy, Carotid"/AE]	115
#45	#28 or #43 or #44	339
#46	harm or harms or adverse effect* or adverse event* or complication* or death or stroke or [mh "Myocardial Infarction"] or "myocardial infarction" or (unnecessary and "carotid endarterectomy") or [mh "Kidney Failure, Chronic"] or [mh "Renal Insufficiency"] or [mh "Cranial Nerve Diseases"] or [mh "Cranial Nerve Injuries"] or (neck and hematoma*)	237643
#47	#45 and #46	310
#48	comment:pt or editorial:pt or letter:pt or news:pt	6431
#49	#33 not #48	233
#50	#40 not #48	109
#51	#42 not #48	12
#52	#47 not #48	308
#53	#49 or #50 or #51 or #52 from 2012 to 2013	**20**

9/27/13 Gray Literature Updates

ClinicalTrials.gov yielded 6 results

("Mass Screening" OR screening OR Ultrasonography OR "carotid endarterectomy" OR Angioplasty OR "Magnetic Resonance Angiography" OR "balloon angioplasty" OR "balloon dilation" OR stent* OR "CT angiography" OR "computed tomographic angiography" OR radiography) [ALL-FIELDS] AND (("carotid stenosis" OR "carotid artery stenosis" AND asymptomatic) AND ("01/12/2013" : "09/27/2013") [FIRST-RECEIVED-DATE]) [ALL-FIELDS]

Appendix B. Search Strategy

Cochrane Trials Search (2 of the 3 results were trials and were saved, but both were duplicates with other update searches [the main Cochrane library update above].)

ID	Search	Hits
#1	[mh "Carotid Stenosis"] or "carotid stenosis" or "carotid artery stenosis"	853
#2	asymptomatic	5772
#3	#1 and #2	268
#4	[mh "Mass Screening"]	4548
#5	#3 and #4	7
#6	[mh "Carotid Stenosis"/US]	112
#7	[mh Ultrasonography]	6996
#8	#3 and #7	48
#9	[mh "Endarterectomy, Carotid"]	461
#10	#3 and #9	129
#11	[mh Angioplasty]	4239
#12	#3 and #11	38
#13	[mh "Magnetic Resonance Angiography"]	350
#14	#3 and #13	5
#15	[mh "Angioplasty, Balloon"] or "balloon dilation"	4026
#16	#3 and #15	19
#17	[mh Stents]	3110
#18	#3 and #17	54
#19	"CT angiography" or "computed tomographic angiography"	275
#20	#3 and #19	3
#21	[mh "Carotid Stenosis"/RA]	53
#22	#3 and #21	11
#23	#5 or #6 or #8 or #10 or #12 or #14 or #16 or #18 or #20 or #22	253
#24	[mh Aspirin] or [mh "Hydroxymethylglutaryl-CoA Reductase Inhibitors"] or (statins:ti or statins:ab) or [mh "Platelet Aggregation Inhibitors"] or [mh "Drug Therapy"] or [mh /DT]	204690
#25	#3 and #24	38
#26	[mh "Pharmacologic Actions"]	160591
#27	#3 and #26	25
#28	#27 not #25	3
#29	#23 or #28	255
#30	comment:pt or editoral:pt or letter:pt or news:pt	6273
#31	#29 not #30 from 2013 to 2013	3

9/27/13 WHO ICTRP (*International Clinical Trials Registry Platform*) Search Update

1) **0** results for Title search: "carotid stenosis" OR "carotid artery stenosis" limited to trials with registry dates between 12/01/2013 - 27/09/2013

2) **0** results for Condition search: "carotid stenosis" OR "carotid artery stenosis" limited to trials with registry dates between 12/01/2013 - 27/09/2013

4/24/2014 Targeted MEDLINE Update Search

Search	Query	Items found
#1	Search ("Carotid Stenosis"[Mesh] OR "carotid stenosis" OR "carotid artery stenosis")	14210
#2	Search asymptomatic	108605
#3	Search (#1 and #2)	2859
#4	Search "Mass Screening"[Mesh]	98103
#5	Search (#3 and #4)	56
#6	Search "Carotid Stenosis/ultrasonography"[Mesh]	2424
#7	Search "Ultrasonography"[Mesh]	244873
#8	Search (#3 and #7)	628
#9	Search "Endarterectomy, Carotid"[Mesh]	6674
#10	Search (#3 and #9)	1213
#11	Search "Angioplasty"[Mesh]	53821

Appendix B. Search Strategy

#12	Search (#3 and #11)	476
#13	Search "Magnetic Resonance Angiography"[Mesh]	16545
#14	Search (#3 and #13)	94
#15	Search ("Angioplasty, Balloon"[Mesh] OR "balloon dilation")	49374
#16	Search (#3 and #15)	236
#17	Search "Stents"[Mesh]	51808
#18	Search (#3 and #17)	651
#19	Search ("CT angiography"[tiab] OR "computed tomographic angiography"[tiab])	7542
#20	Search (#3 and #19)	38
#21	Search "Carotid Stenosis/radiography"[Mesh]	1711
#22	Search (#3 and #21)	250
#23	Search (#5 or #6 or #8 or #10 or #12 or #14 or #16 or #18 or #20 or #22)	4028
#24	Search ("Randomized Controlled Trial"[Publication Type] OR "Single-Blind Method"[MeSH] OR "Double-Blind Method"[MeSH] OR "Random Allocation"[MeSH] OR trial[tiab])	670734
#25	Search (#23 and #24)	471
#26	Search ("review"[Publication Type] AND "systematic"[tiab]) OR "systematic review"[All Fields] OR ("review literature as topic"[MeSH] AND "systematic"[tiab]) OR "meta-analysis"[Publication Type] OR "meta-analysis as topic"[MeSH Terms] OR "meta-analysis"[All Fields])	125426
#27	Search (#23 and #26)	77
#28	Search (#25 or #27)	529
#29	Search ("stroke"[MeSH Terms] OR "stroke"[All Fields] OR "brain infarction"[All Fields] OR "cerebrovascular disorder"[All Fields] OR "cerebrovascular disease"[All Fields] OR "CVA"[All Fields] OR "cerebral infarction"[All Fields] OR "ischemic stroke"[All Fields] OR (("stroke"[MeSH Terms] OR "stroke"[All Fields]) AND ("ischemia"[MeSH Terms] OR "ischemia"[All Fields] OR "ischemic"[All Fields])) OR "cerebrovascular accident"[All Fields])	224012
#30	Search ("risk"[MeSH Terms] OR "risk assessment"[MeSH Terms] OR "risk adjustment"[MeSH Terms] OR "risk assessment"[MeSH Terms] OR ("risk"[All Fields] AND "assessment"[All Fields]) OR "risk assessment"[All Fields] OR ("assessment"[All Fields] AND "benefit"[All Fields] AND "risk"[All Fields]) OR ("assessments"[All Fields] AND "benefit"[All Fields] AND "risk"[All Fields]))	878928
#31	Search (#3 and #29 and #30)	884
#32	Search (#31 and #24)	141
#33	Search ("Case-Control Studies"[MeSH] OR "Cohort Studies"[MeSH] OR "comparative study"[pt] OR "Epidemiologic Studies"[MeSH] OR "Cross-Over Studies"[MeSH] OR "Follow-Up Studies"[MeSH] OR "observational study" OR "observational studies" OR "cohort"[tw] OR "case control"[tw])	3108166
#34	Search (#31 and #33)	524
#35	Search (#32 or #34)	567
#36	Search (#5 or #6 or #8 or #14 or #20 or #22)	2935
#37	Search (#36 and #26)	30
#38	Search ("Endarterectomy, Carotid/statistics and numerical data"[Mesh])	844
#39	Search "Endarterectomy, Carotid/adverse effects"[Mesh]	1715
#40	Search (#23 or #38 or #39)	5681
#41	Search (harm OR harms OR adverse effect* OR adverse event* OR complication* OR death OR stroke OR "Myocardial Infarction"[Mesh] OR "myocardial infarction" OR (unnecessary AND "carotid endarterectomy") OR "Kidney Failure, Chronic"[Mesh] OR "Renal Insufficiency"[Mesh] OR "Cranial Nerve Diseases"[Mesh] OR "Cranial Nerve Injuries"[Mesh] OR (neck AND hematoma*))	4190723
#42	Search (#40 and #41)	4378
#43	Search (comment[pt] OR editorial[pt] OR letter[pt] OR news[pt])	1458299
#44	Search (#25 or #27) Filters: Humans	526
#45	Search (#25 or #27) Filters: Humans; English	489
#46	Search (#25 or #27) Filters: Humans; English; Adult: 19+ years	303
#47	Search (#46 NOT #43)	303
#48	Search (#32 or #34) Filters: Humans	566
#49	Search (#32 or #34) Filters: Humans; English	527
#50	Search (#32 or #34) Filters: Humans; English; Adult: 19+ years	453
#51	Search (#50 NOT #43)	452
#52	Search (#36 and #26) Filters: Humans	30
#53	Search (#36 and #26) Filters: Humans; English	28

Appendix B. Search Strategy

#54	Search (#36 and #26) Filters: Humans; English; Adult: 19+ years	8
#55	Search (#54 NOT #43)	8
#56	Search (#40 and #41) Filters: Humans	4354
#57	Search (#40 and #41) Filters: Humans; English	3928
#58	Search (#40 and #41) Filters: Humans; English; Adult: 19+ years	2804
#59	Search (#58 NOT #43)	2745
#60	Search (#47 or #51 or #55 or #59)	2870
#61	Search (#60 AND (2013/03/01:2014/03/31[edat]))	**81**
#62	Search (#21 or #31 or #42)	5889
#63	Search (#62 AND ("retraction"[All Fields] OR "Retracted Publication"[pt]))	**3**

Search	Query	Items found
#1	Search ("Carotid Stenosis"[Mesh] OR "carotid stenosis" OR "carotid artery stenosis")	14210
#2	Search asymptomatic	108605
#3	Search (#1 and #2)	2859
#4	Search ("Aspirin"[Mesh] OR "Hydroxymethylglutaryl-CoA Reductase Inhibitors" [Pharmacological Action] OR "Hydroxymethylglutaryl-CoA Reductase Inhibitors" [Mesh] OR statins[tiab] OR "Platelet Aggregation Inhibitors"[Mesh] OR "Drug Therapy"[Mesh] OR "drug therapy"[subheading])	2273767
#5	Search (#3 and #4)	257
#6	Search ("Chemicals and Drugs Category"[Mesh])	11386211
#7	Search (#3 and #6)	548
#8	Search (#7 NOT #5)	344
#9	Search ("Randomized Controlled Trial"[Publication Type] OR "Single-Blind Method"[MeSH] OR "Double-Blind Method"[MeSH] OR "Random Allocation"[MeSH] OR trial[tiab])	670734
#10	Search (#8 and #9)	20
#11	Search (#8 and #9) Filters: Humans	20
#12	Search (#8 and #9) Filters: Humans; English	17
#13	Search (#8 and #9) Filters: Humans; English; Adult: 19+ years	15
#14	Search ("review"[Publication Type] AND "systematic"[tiab]) OR "systematic review"[All Fields] OR ("review literature as topic"[MeSH] AND "systematic"[tiab]) OR "meta-analysis"[Publication Type] OR "meta-analysis as topic"[MeSH Terms] OR "meta-analysis"[All Fields])) Filters: Humans; English; Adult: 19+ years	21895
#15	Search (#8 and #14) Filters: Humans; English; Adult: 19+ years	0
#16	Search (Chlorthalidone[mesh] AND #8)	0
#17	Search (Chlorthalidone[mesh] AND #3)	0
#18	Search (Hydrochlorothiazide[mesh] AND #3)	3
#19	Search (#18 AND (#9 or #14))	3
#20	Search (#18 AND (#9 or #14)) Filters: Humans	3
#21	Search (#18 AND (#9 or #14)) Filters: Humans; English	3
#22	Search (#18 AND (#9 or #14)) Filters: Humans; English; Adult: 19+ years	3
#23	Search (#22 NOT (#5 or #13)) Filters: Humans; English; Adult: 19+ years	0
#24	Search ("Lisinopril"[Mesh] AND #3) Filters: Humans; English; Adult: 19+ years	0
#25	Search ("Metoprolol"[Mesh] AND #3) Filters: Humans; English; Adult: 19+ years	0
#26	Search (#5 and (#9 or #14)) Filters: Humans; English; Adult: 19+ years	46
#27	Search (#13 or #22 or #26) Filters: Humans; English; Adult: 19+ years	61
#28	Search (#13 or #22 or #26)	61
#29	Search (#27 AND (2013/03/01:2014/03/31[edat])) Filters: Humans; English; Adult: 19+ years	4
#30	Search ((#5 or #7 or #18) AND ("retraction"[All Fields] OR "Retracted Publication"[pt]))	0

Appendix B Table 1. Inclusion and Exclusion Criteria

	Inclusion	Exclusion
Populations	Asymptomatic adults with CAS that is potentially clinically important (defined as 60% to 99% stenosis). Asymptomatic indicates that patients have no significant neurologic symptoms referable to the carotid artery and have not experienced a cerebrovascular event (i.e., a stroke or transient ischemic attack). We will include studies that enroll both symptomatic and asymptomatic subjects, but that analyze the asymptomatic group separately. Among asymptomatic subjects, some trials enroll a minority of subjects who have not had symptoms for some specified time period (e.g., the past 180 days), but who had prior symptoms or cerebrovascular events. Although our focus is on people who have never had cerebrovascular events, we will include such studies if they enroll 70% or more of subjects who never had symptoms referable to the carotid artery and never had a cerebrovascular event into the "asymptomatic" group.	Children and adolescents; symptomatic adults with CAS; adults with history of transient ischemic attacks or stroke; studies of people with carotid occlusion; studies of people undergoing CABG and others confined to a focused population, such as those with radiation exposure or PVD; people with remote CEA or CAAS undergoing surveillance for restenosis.
Setting	Studies conducted in developed countries.	
Screening	Screening with carotid duplex ultrasonography, used alone or followed by CTA or MRA with or without confirmatory testing with angiography. Studies that use a single screening test as well as those that use multiple tests in series (e.g., ultrasonography followed by MRA for persons with potentially significant ultrasound findings) will be included.	Physical examination for carotid bruit.
Treatment/ management interventions	CEA, CAAS, medical therapy (e.g., aspirin, statins, antiplatelet medications)	
Comparisons	KQ 1: Screened versus nonscreened groups. KQ 2: Studies must determine/compare those at increased, average, or decreased risk, or those at higher and lower risk of CAS of 60% to 99%. KQ 3: Studies on accuracy of screening must include a comparison with angiography; studies on reliability of screening must include measures of reproducibility (e.g., test-retest, comparison between different labs or readers). KQ 4: Studies must determine/compare those at increased, average, or decreased risk, or those at higher and lower risk of ipsilateral stroke (KQ 4a) or periprocedural harms from CEA or CAAS (KQ 4b). KQ 5: Medical treatment/usual care. KQ 6: Studies must compare the addition of one or more medications to current standard medical therapy (that includes treatment of traditional risk factors) versus the addition of placebo to current standard medical therapy (that includes treatment of traditional risk factors). KQ 7: Screened versus nonscreened groups or those having angiography versus not having angiography or noncomparative studies reporting rates of harms. KQ 8: Medical treatment/usual care or noncomparative studies reporting rates of harms.	No comparison; nonconcordant historical controls; comparative studies of CEA versus CAAS.
Outcomes	KQs 1, 5, and 6 (health outcomes): CAS-related fatal or nonfatal stroke. Quality of life and functional status. KQ 2 (assessment of risk stratification tools): Adjusted hazard ratio (or risk ratio or odds ratio), discrimination, calibration, reclassification; tools must be externally validated. KQ 3 (diagnostic accuracy and reliability of screening tests): Sensitivity and specificity. KQ 4 (assessment of risk stratification tools): Adjusted hazard ratio (or risk ratio or odds ratio), discrimination, calibration, reclassification; tools must be externally validated. KQ 7 (harms of screening or confirmatory tests): False positives leading to unnecessary treatment, nonfatal stroke, fatal stroke, persistent neurological complications, renal failure. KQ 8 (harms of CEA or CAAS): Perioperative complications, including stroke, death, nonfatal myocardial infarction, cranial nerve injuries.	Restenosis, quality-adjusted life years.

Appendix B Table 1. Inclusion and Exclusion Criteria

	Inclusion	Exclusion
Study designs	KQ 1: Randomized, controlled trials (RCTs) that compare screened versus nonscreened groups. KQ 2: Cohort studies that develop risk stratification tools and then validate the tools using an external population. Studies must follow a cohort of asymptomatic people to develop a tool, derived from a multivariate analysis, predicting risk of CAS. Risk stratification tools (or "risk prediction tools") must combine multiple variables and allow us to calculate risk for individual patients. KQ 3: Systematic reviews that compare screening tests (ultrasonography, MRA, or CTA) with angiography. Primary studies comparing screening tests with angiography that were published after the included systematic reviews will be included (i.e., bridge searches will be performed to determine what is new since the systematic reviews and whether it is consistent with the systematic reviews). KQ 4: Cohort studies that develop risk stratification tools for adults with asymptomatic CAS and then validate the tools using an external population. Studies must follow a cohort of people with asymptomatic CAS of 60% to 99% to develop a tool, derived from a multivariate analysis, predicting risk of ipsilateral stroke (KQ 4a) or periprocedural harms (KQ 4b). Risk stratification tools (or "risk prediction tools") must combine multiple variables and allow us to calculate risk for individual patients. Risk stratification tools may include clinical factors (e.g., age, diabetes) and anatomic or imaging predictors (e.g., plaque area or morphology, silent embolic events, contralateral disease). KQ 5: Systematic reviews and RCTs of CEA or CAAS comparing surgical/interventional treatment with medical treatment. KQ 6: Systematic reviews and RCTs. KQ 7: Systematic reviews or multi-institution studies (RCTs or cohort studies) that report harms of screening or confirmatory tests. KQ 8: Systematic reviews or multi-institution studies (RCTs or cohort studies) that report 30-day or longer harms for asymptomatic patients undergoing CEA or CAAS.	All other designs; studies enrolling both symptomatic and asymptomatic patients that don't analyze them separately.
Language	English	Non-English

Note: For the population of interest, we will not rigidly consider those with 60% to 99% CAS as a single homogeneous cohort. Rather, we will include studies enrolling participants beyond that degree of CAS (e.g., 50% to 99% CAS), and we will evaluate the available evidence for various subgroups within that cohort. For example, we will evaluate evidence for those with 80% to 99% CAS, if available.

The settings are limited to developed countries to find evidence most applicable to the United States. Other settings are unlikely to have screening and interventions comparable to those in the United States.

Physical examination for carotid bruit is not included as a screening method under evaluation because an earlier review for the USPSTF (1996) concluded that auscultation for carotid bruits is imperfect, with low sensitivity and specificity and considerable interobserver variation in the interpretation of key auditory characteristics. We scanned the literature published since the 1996 review and found no compelling evidence to suggest that auscultation has become any better as a screening tool to detect clinically significant levels of asymptomatic CAS. Our search identified 51 references, of which 4 reported on the accuracy of screening for CAS by auscultation of the carotid artery. Those studies used varying cutoffs for CAS; minimum cutoff values ranged from 50% to 70%. All studies used ultrasound as the gold standard. The reported sensitivities ranged from 46% to 77%, and specificities ranged from 71% to 98%. Notably, only 2 of the studies were of patients from the general population (one in the United States and the other in France); one study included Swedish patients referred to a hospital for carotid surgery investigation, and the fourth study was among Chinese patients with peripheral vascular disease.

Appendix C. Excluded Studies

Not Original Research

1. Power Doppler detects stroke risk in patients without stenosis symptoms. Geriatrics. 2000;55(8):15-22.
2. Barnett HJ, Meldrum HE. The outlook for patients with carotid stenosis. Cerebrovasc Dis. 2000;10(Suppl 4):30-5. PMID: 11070398.
3. Hankey GJ. Carotid endarterectomy for asymptomatic carotid stenosis. Ann Intern Med. 1993;118(Suppl 3):72.
4. Khan N, Murphy TP, Haas RA, et al. Stroke prevention. Med Health R I. 2005;88(2):44-7. PMID: 15816244.
5. Meissner I. Symptomatic carotid stenosis: precarotid endarterectomy evaluation. J Neurosurg Anesthesiol. 1996;8(4):308-9. PMID: 8884629.
6. Newell DW, Grady MS, Nicholls SC. Cervical carotid to petrous carotid bypass for lesions of the upper cervical carotid artery. Ann Vasc Surg. 1996;10(1):76-87.
7. Sacco RL. Extracranial carotid stenosis. N Engl J Med. 2001;345(15):1113-8.
8. Towne JB, Hobson RW. Current status of operative treatment for asymptomatic carotid stenosis. Can J Surg. 1994;37(2):128-34. PMID: 8156465.

Ineligible Population

1. AbuRahma AF, Bates MC, Eads K, et al. Safety and efficacy of carotid angioplasty/stenting in 100 consecutive high surgical risk patients: immediate and long-term follow-up. Vasc Endovascular Surg. 2008;42(5):433-9. PMID: 18583300.
2. Ackerstaff RG, Moons KG, van de Vlasakker CJ, et al. Association of intraoperative transcranial doppler monitoring variables with stroke from carotid endarterectomy. Stroke. 2000;31(8):1817-23. PMID: 10926940.
3. Ahari A, Bergqvist D, Troeng T, et al. Diabetes mellitus as a risk factor for early outcome after carotid endarterectomy--a population-based study. Eur J Vasc Endovasc Surg. 1999;18(2):122-6. PMID: 10428751.
4. Alexandrova NA, Gibson WC, Norris JW, et al. Carotid artery stenosis in peripheral vascular disease. J Vasc Surg. 1996;23(4):645-9. PMID: 8627901.
5. Amato B, Markabaoui AK, Piscitelli V, et al. Carotid endarterectomy under local anesthesia in elderly: is it worthwhile? Acta Biomed. 2005;76(Suppl 1):64-8. PMID: 16450515.
6. Aoki J, Kimura K, Iguchi Y, et al. A combined TCD and MRA screening for significant siphon portion of internal carotid artery (S-ICA) stenosis. J Neuroimaging. 2012;22(2):172-6. PMID: 21223433.
7. Beilby JP, Hunt CC, Palmer LJ, et al. Apolipoprotein E gene polymorphisms are associated with carotid plaque formation but not with intima-media wall thickening: results from the Perth Carotid Ultrasound Disease Assessment Study (CUDAS). Stroke. 2003;34(4):869-74. PMID: 12637699.
8. Biasi GM, Froio A, Diethrich EB, et al. Carotid plaque echolucency increases the risk of stroke in carotid stenting: the Imaging in Carotid Angioplasty and Risk of Stroke (ICAROS) study. Circulation. 2004;110(6):756-62. PMID: 15277320.
9. Bonati Leo H, Lyrer P, Ederle J, et al. Percutaneous transluminal balloon angioplasty and stenting for carotid artery stenosis. Cochrane Database Syst Rev: John Wiley & Sons, Ltd; 2012.
10. Bond R, Narayan SK, Rothwell PM, et al. Clinical and radiographic risk factors for operative stroke and death in the European carotid surgery trial. Eur J Vasc Endovasc Surg. 2002;23(2):108-16. PMID: 11863327.
11. Bond R, Rerkasem K, Cuffe R, et al. A systematic review of the associations between age and sex and the operative risks of carotid endarterectomy. Cerebrovasc Dis. 2005;20(2):69-77. PMID: 15976498.
12. Borisch I, Horn M, Butz B, et al. Preoperative evaluation of carotid artery stenosis: comparison of contrast-enhanced MR angiography and duplex sonography with digital subtraction angiography. Am J Neuroradiol. 2003;24(6):1117-22.
13. Bosiers M, De Donato G, Deloose K, et al. Are there predictive risk factors for complications after carotid artery stenting? J Cardiovasc Surg (Torino). 2007;48(2):125-30. PMID: 17410060.
14. Bots ML, van Swieten JC, Breteler MM, et al. Cerebral white matter lesions and atherosclerosis in the Rotterdam Study. Lancet. 1993;341(8855):1232-7. PMID: 8098390.
15. Brown HA, Sullivan MC, Gusberg RG, Dardik A, Sosa JA, Indes JE. Race as a predictor of morbidity, mortality, and neurologic events after carotid endarterectomy. J Vasc Surg. 2013;57(5):1325-1330.
16. Bush RL, Kougias P, Guerrero MA, et al. A comparison of carotid artery stenting with neuroprotection versus carotid endarterectomy under local anesthesia. Am J Surg. 2005;190(5):696-700. PMID: 16226942.
17. Cao P, De Rango P, Zannetti S. Eversion vs conventional carotid endarterectomy: a systematic review. Eur J Vasc Endovasc Surg. 2002;23(3):195-201. PMID: 11914004.

Appendix C. Excluded Studies

18. Carmody BJ, Arora S, Avena R, et al. Accelerated carotid artery disease after high-dose head and neck radiotherapy: is there a role for routine carotid duplex surveillance? J Vasc Surg. 1999;30(6):1045-51. PMID: 10587388.

19. Chang JB, Stein TA. Late stroke in patients after carotid endarterectomy. J Surg Res. 1997;73(2):155-9. PMID: 9441810.

20. Chang JB, Stein TA. Ten-year outcome after saphenous vein patch angioplasty in males and females after carotid endarterectomy. Vasc Endovascular Surg. 2002;36(1):21-7. PMID: 12704521.

21. Collins P, McKay I, Rajagoplan S, et al. Is carotid duplex scanning sufficient as the sole investigation prior to carotid endarterectomy? Br J Radiol. 2005;78(935):1034-7. PMID: 16249605.

22. Dean N, Lari H, Saqqur M, et al. Reliability of carotid doppler performed in a dedicated stroke prevention clinic. Can J Neurol Sci. 2005;32(3):327-31. PMID: 16225174.

23. Debing E, Van den Brande P. Does the type, number or combinations of traditional cardiovascular risk factors affect early outcome after carotid endarterectomy? Eur J Vasc Endovasc Surg. 2006;31(6):622-6. PMID: 16466942.

24. Droste DW, Jurgens R, Weber S, et al. Benefit of echocontrast-enhanced transcranial color-coded duplex ultrasound in the assessment of intracranial collateral pathways. Stroke. 2000;31(4):920-3. PMID: 10753999.

25. Duncan JM, Reul GJ, Ott DA, et al. Outcomes and risk factors in 1,609 carotid endarterectomies. Tex Heart Inst J. 2008;35(2):104-10. PMID: 18612484.

26. Endo S, Kuwayama N, Hirashima Y. Japan Carotid Atherosclerosis Study: JCAS. Neurol Med Chir (Tokyo). 2004;44(4):215-7.

27. Engelhardt M, Bruijnen H, Schnur C, et al. Duplex scanning criteria for selection of patients for internal carotid artery endarterectomy. Vasa. 2005;34(1):36-40. PMID: 15786936.

28. Engelter S, Lyrer P. Antiplatelet therapy for preventing stroke and other vascular events after carotid endarterectomy. Cochrane Database Syst Rev: John Wiley & Sons, Ltd; 2003.

29. Fabris F, Zanocchi M, Bo M, et al. Carotid plaque, aging, and risk factors. A study of 457 subjects. Stroke. 1994;25(6):1133-40. PMID: 8202970.

30. Flis V, Tetickovic E, Breznik S, et al. The measurement of stenosis of the internal carotid artery: comparison of doppler ultrasound, digital subtraction angiography and the 3D CT volume rendering technique. Wien Klin Wochenschr. 2004;116(Suppl 2):51-5. PMID: 15506311.

31. Florio F, Nardella M, Balzano S, et al. Preoperative assessment of stenosis of the epiaortic vessels: can colour-Doppler ultrasound really supplant angiography? Radiol Med. 2003;105(4):362-9. PMID: 12835630.

32. Fujimoto S, Toyoda K, Kishikawa K, et al. Accuracy of conventional plus transoral carotid ultrasonography in distinguishing pseudo-occlusion from total occlusion of the internal carotid artery. Cerebrovasc Dis. 2006;22(2-3):170-6.

33. Gabrusiewicz A, Staszkiewicz W, Slowinski P, et al. Clinical assessment of the factors influencing neurological deficits during carotid endarterectomy. Chirurgia Polska. 2007;9(2):69-77.

34. Gao MY, Sillesen HH, Lorentzen JE, et al. Eversion carotid endarterectomy generates fewer microemboli than standard carotid endarterectomy. Eur J Vasc Endovasc Surg. 2000;20(2):153-7. PMID: 10942686.

35. Goodney PP, Likosky DS, Cronenwett JL. Factors associated with stroke or death after carotid endarterectomy in Northern New England. J Vasc Surg. 2008;48(5):1139-45. PMID: 18586446.

36. Grego F, Lepidi S, Antonello M, et al. Is carotid endarterectomy in octogenarians more dangerous than in younger patients? J Cardiovasc Surg (Torino). 2005;46(5):477-83. PMID: 16278638.

37. Griewing B, Brassel F, Von Smekal U, et al. Carotid artery stenting in patients at surgical high risk: clinical and ultrasound findings. Cerebrovasc Dis. 2000;10(1):44-8.

38. Gupta PK, Pipinos II, Miller WJ, et al. A population-based study of risk factors for stroke after carotid endarterectomy using the ACS NSQIP database. J Surg Res. 2011;167(2):182-91. PMID: 21109261.

39. Hart JP, Peeters P, Verbist J, et al. Do device characteristics impact outcome in carotid artery stenting? J Vasc Surg. 2006;44(4):725-30. PMID: 17011998.

40. Harthun NL, Kongable GL, Baglioni AJ, et al. Examination of sex as an independent risk factor for adverse events after carotid endarterectomy. J Vasc Surg. 2005;41(2):223-30. PMID: 15768003.

41. Hashimoto H, Tagaya M, Niki H, et al. Computer-assisted analysis of heterogeneity on B-mode imaging predicts instability of asymptomatic carotid plaque. Cerebrovasc Dis. 2009;28(4):357-64. PMID: 19628937.

42. Hayes PD, Allroggen H, Steel S, et al. Randomized trial of vein versus Dacron patching during carotid endarterectomy: influence of patch type on postoperative embolization. J Vasc Surg. 2001;33(5):994-1000. PMID: 11331840.

43. Helm EE. Clinical and operative predictors of outcomes of carotid endarterectomy. J Vasc Surg. 2005;42(3).

Appendix C. Excluded Studies

44. Henry M, Henry I, Polydorou A, et al. Carotid angioplasty and stenting in octogenarians: is it safe? Catheter Cardiovasc Interv. 2008;72(3):309-17. PMID: 18729151.
45. Henry MC, Henry I, Benjelloun A. Carotid angioplasty and stenting in octogenarians is as safe as surgery. Heart Surg Forum. 2012;15:S51-S2.
46. Herzig R, Burval S, Krupka B, et al. Comparison of ultrasonography, CT angiography, and digital subtraction angiography in severe carotid stenoses. Eur J Neurol. 2004;11(11):774-81.
47. Heyer EJ, Wilson DA, Sahlein DH, et al. APOE-ε4 predisposes to cognitive dysfunction following uncomplicated carotid endarterectomy. Neurology. 2005;65(11):1759-63. PMID: 16207841.
48. Hsia DC, Moscoe LM, Krushat WM. Epidemiology of carotid endarterectomy among Medicare beneficiaries: 1985-1996 update. Stroke. 1998;29(2):346-50. PMID: 9472872.
49. Jackson RS, Black JH 3rd, Lum YW, et al. Class I obesity is paradoxically associated with decreased risk of postoperative stroke after carotid endarterectomy. J Vasc Surg. 2012;55(5):1306-12. PMID: 22542344.
50. Jung EM, Kubale R, Ritter G, et al. Diagnostics and characterisation of preocclusive stenoses and occlusions of the internal carotid artery with B-flow. Eur Radiol. 2007;17(2):439-47.
51. Katz SG, Kohl RD. Does the choice of material influence early morbidity in patients undergoing carotid patch angioplasty? Surgery. 1996;119(3):297-301. PMID: 8619185.
52. Kerdiles Y, Lucas A, Podeur L, et al. Results of carotid surgery in elderly patients. J Cardiovasc Surg (Torino). 1997;38(4):327-34. PMID: 9267339.
53. Kimouli M, Miyakis S, Georgakopoulos P, et al. Polymorphisms of fractalkine receptor CX3CR1 gene in patients with symptomatic and asymptomatic carotid artery stenosis. J Atheroscler Thromb. 2009;16(5):604-10.
54. Koelemay ME. Systematic review of computed tomographic angiography for assessment of carotid artery disease. Stroke. 2004;35(10).
55. Kragsterman B, Logason K, Ahari A, et al. Risk factors for complications after carotid endarterectomy--a population-based study. Eur J Vasc Endovasc Surg. 2004;28(1):98-103. PMID: 15177238.
56. Kucey DS, Bowyer B, Iron K, et al. Determinants of outcome after carotid endarterectomy. J Vasc Surg. 1998;28(6):1051-8. PMID: 9845656.
57. Kueh SH, Livingstone V, Thomson IA. Carotid endarterectomy in octogenarians. N Z Med J. 2012;125(1364):77-82.
58. Kuhan G, Gardiner ED, Abidia AF, et al. Risk modelling study for carotid endarterectomy. Br J Surg. 2001;88(12):1590-4. PMID: 11736969.
59. Kuntz KM, Polak JF, Whittemore AD, et al. Duplex ultrasound criteria for the identification of carotid stenosis should be laboratory specific. Stroke. 1997;28(3):597-602. PMID: 9056618.
60. Lawrence PF, Alves JC, Jicha D, et al. Incidence, timing, and causes of cerebral ischemia during carotid endarterectomy with regional anesthesia. J Vasc Surg. 1998;27(2):329-34. PMID: 9510287.
61. Lennard N, Smith JL, Gaunt ME, et al. A policy of quality control assessment helps to reduce the risk of intraoperative stroke during carotid endarterectomy. Eur J Vasc Endovasc Surg. 1999;17(3):234-40. PMID: 10092897.
62. Lernfelt B, Forsberg M, Blomstrand C, et al. Cerebral atherosclerosis as predictor of stroke and mortality in representative elderly population. Stroke. 2002;33(1):224-9. PMID: 11779914.
63. Liapis CD, Kakisis JD, Papavassiliou VG, et al. Risk factors associated with recurrent carotid artery stenosis. Vasc Surg. 1999;33(6):697-704.
64. Lindgren A, Roijer A, Rudling O, et al. Cerebral lesions on magnetic resonance imaging, heart disease, and vascular risk factors in subjects without stroke. A population-based study. Stroke. 1994;25(5):929-34. PMID: 8165686.
65. Logason K, Karacagil S, Hardemark HG, et al. Carotid artery endarterectomy solely based on duplex scan findings. Vasc Surg. 2002;36(1):9-15.
66. Lopez-Cancio E, Dorado L, Millan M, et al. The Barcelona-Asymptomatic Intracranial Atherosclerosis (AsIA) study: prevalence and risk factors. Atherosclerosis. 2012;221(1):221-5.
67. Lyrer P, Engelter S. Antithrombotic drugs for carotid artery dissection. Cochrane Database Syst Rev: John Wiley & Sons, Ltd; 2010.
68. Madycki G, Staszkiewicz W, Gabrusiewicz A. Carotid plaque texture analysis can predict the incidence of silent brain infarcts among patients undergoing carotid endarterectomy. Eur J Vasc Endovasc Surg. 2006;31(4):373-80. PMID: 16427334.
69. Manheim LM, Sohn MW, Feinglass J, et al. Hospital vascular surgery volume and procedure mortality rates in California, 1982-1994. J Vasc Surg. 1998;28(1):45-56. PMID: 9685130.

Appendix C. Excluded Studies

70. Mathiesen EB, Bonaa KH, Joakimsen O. Echolucent plaques are associated with high risk of ischemic cerebrovascular events in carotid stenosis: the Tromso study. Circulation. 2001;103(17):2171-5. PMID: 11331258.

71. Matsen SL, Perler BA, Chang DC. A preliminary clinical scale to predict the risk of in-hospital death after carotid endarterectomy. J Vasc Surg. 2005;42(5):861-8. PMID: 16275438.

72. Mauney MC, Buchanan SA, Lawrence WA, et al. Stroke rate is markedly reduced after carotid endarterectomy by avoidance of protamine. J Vasc Surg. 1995;22(3):264-9. PMID: 7674469.

73. McBrien K, Rabi DM, Campbell N, et al. Intensive and standard blood pressure targets in patients with type 2 diabetes mellitus: systematic review and meta-analysis. Arch Intern Med. 2012;172(17):1296-303. PMID: 22868819.

74. McKevitt FM, Sivaguru A, Venables GS, et al. Effect of treatment of carotid artery stenosis on blood pressure: a comparison of hemodynamic disturbances after carotid endarterectomy and endovascular treatment. Stroke. 2003;34(11):2576-81. PMID: 14593127.

75. Messe SR, Kasner SE, Mehta Z, et al. Effect of body size on operative risk of carotid endarterectomy. J Neurol Neurosurg Psychiatry. 2004;75(12):1759-61. PMID: 15548500.

76. Mingoli A, Sapienza P, Feldhaus RJ, et al. Carotid endarterectomy in young adults: is it a worthwhile procedure? J Vasc Surg. 1997;25(3):464-70. PMID: 9081127.

77. Mocco J, Wilson DA, Komotar RJ, et al. Galbraith Award: evaluation of risk factors associated with neurocognitive changes after carotid endarterectomy. Clin Neurosurg. 2006;53:301-6. PMID: 17380766.

78. Mocco J, Wilson DA, Komotar RJ, et al. Predictors of neurocognitive decline after carotid endarterectomy. Neurosurgery. 2006;58(5):844-50. PMID: 16639318.

79. Mommertz G, Das M, Langer S, et al. Early control of distal internal carotid artery during carotid endarterectomy: does it reduce cerebral microemboli? J Cardiovasc Surg (Torino). 2010;51(3):369-75. PMID: 20523287.

80. Naylor R, Hayes PD, Payne DA, et al. Randomized trial of vein versus Dacron patching during carotid endarterectomy: long-term results. J Vasc Surg. 2004;39(5):985-93.

81. Pieniazek P, Musialek P, Kablak-Ziembicka A, et al. Carotid artery stenting with patient- and lesion-tailored selection of the neuroprotection system and stent type: early and 5-year results from a prospective academic registry of 535 consecutive procedures (TARGET-CAS). J Endovasc Ther. 2008;15(3):249-62. PMID: 18540694.

82. Polak JF, Szklo M, Kronmal RA, et al. The value of carotid artery plaque and intima-media thickness for incident cardiovascular disease: the multi-ethnic study of atherosclerosis. J Am Heart Assoc. 2013;2(2):e000087.

83. Qureshi AI, Suri MF, New G, et al. Multicenter study of the feasibility and safety of using the memotherm carotid arterial stent for extracranial carotid artery stenosis. J Neurosurg. 2002;96(5):830-6. PMID: 12005390.

84. Revnic CR, Prada GI, Pena C, et al. Evaluation of total serum MMP-9 and their inhibitors TIMP-1 as a markers of carotid plaque instability in elderly patients with carotid stenosis. Eur J Neurol. 2012;19:181.

85. Robertson L, Ghouri Maaz A, Kovacs F. Antiplatelet and anticoagulant drugs for prevention of restenosis/reocclusion following peripheral endovascular treatment. Cochrane Database Syst Rev: John Wiley & Sons, Ltd; 2012.

86. Saba L, Sanfilippo R, Anzidei M, et al. Stenosis Asymmetry Index (SAI) between symptomatic and asymptomatic patients in the analysis of carotid arteries. A study using CT angiography. Eur J Radiol. 2012;81(1):77-82. PMID: 21242044.

87. Sabeti S, Schlager O, Exner M, et al. Progression of carotid stenosis detected by duplex ultrasonography predicts adverse outcomes in cardiovascular high-risk patients. Stroke. 2007;38(11):2887-94. PMID: 17885257.

88. Sadato A, Satow T, Ishii A, et al. Use of a large angioplasty balloon for predilation is a risk factor for embolic complications in protected carotid stenting. Neurol Med Chir (Tokyo). 2004;44(7):337-42. PMID: 15347209.

89. Sameshima T, Futami S, Morita Y, et al. Clinical usefulness of and problems with three-dimensional CT angiography for the evaluation of arteriosclerotic stenosis of the carotid artery: comparison with conventional angiography, MRA, and ultrasound sonography. Surg Neurol. 1999;51(3):301-8. PMID: 10086495.

90. Sandercock PA, Counsell C, Kamal Ayeesha K. Anticoagulants for acute ischaemic stroke. Cochrane Database Syst Rev: John Wiley & Sons, Ltd; 2008.

91. Sayeed S, Stanziale SF, Wholey MH, et al. Angiographic lesion characteristics can predict adverse outcomes after carotid artery stenting. J Vasc Surg. 2008;47(1):81-7. PMID: 18178457.

92. Scavee V, Theys S, Schoevaerdts JC. Does retrojugular route for carotid endarterectomy increase the risk of internal jugular vein thrombosis? Acta Chir Belg. 2006;106(4):397-9. PMID: 17017691.

Appendix C. Excluded Studies

93. Self DD, Bryson GL, Sullivan PJ. Risk factors for post-carotid endarterectomy hematoma formation. Can J Anaesth. 1999;46(7):635-40. PMID: 10442957.
94. Seretis K, Goudakos I, Vlachakis I, et al. Carotid artery disease in octogenarians: endarterectomy or stenting? (Structured abstract). Int Angiol. 2007:353-60.
95. Sheikh K, Bullock C. Variation and changes in state-specific carotid endarterectomy and 30-day mortality rates, United States, 1991-2000. J Vasc Surg. 2003;38(4):779-84. PMID: 14560230.
96. Silvestrini M, Troisi E, Matteis M, et al. Transcranial Doppler assessment of cerebrovascular reactivity in symptomatic and asymptomatic severe carotid stenosis. Stroke. 1996;27(11):1970-3. PMID: 8898800.
97. Simons JP, Goodney PP, Baril DT, et al. The effect of postoperative stroke and myocardial infarction on long-term survival after carotid revascularization. J Vasc Surg. 2013;57(6):1581-8.
98. Slovut DP, Romero JM, Hannon KM, et al. Detection of common carotid artery stenosis using duplex ultrasonography: a validation study with computed tomographic angiography. J Vasc Surg. 2010;51(1):65-70. PMID: 19879097.
99. Staub D, Patel MB, Tibrewala A, et al. Vasa vasorum and plaque neovascularization on contrast-enhanced carotid ultrasound imaging correlates with cardiovascular disease and past cardiovascular events. Stroke. 2010;41(1):41-7. PMID: 19910551.
100. Steinberg J. Does carotid endarterectomy benefit patients with carotid stenosis but no symptoms? J Fam Pract. 2000;49(7):600, 55. PMID: 10923567.
101. Sudlow CL, Mason G, Maurice James B, et al. Thienopyridine derivatives versus aspirin for preventing stroke and other serious vascular events in high vascular risk patients. Cochrane Database Syst Rev: John Wiley & Sons, Ltd; 2009.
102. Takach TJ, Reul GJ Jr, Cooley DA, et al. Is an integrated approach warranted for concomitant carotid and coronary artery disease? Ann Thorac Surg. 1997;64(1):16-22. PMID: 9236329.
103. Taniguchi N, Itoh K, Honda M, et al. Comparative ultrasonographic and angiographic study of carotid arterial lesions in Takayasu's arteritis. Angiology. 1997;48(1):9-20. PMID: 8995338.
104. Telman G, Kouperberg E, Sprecher E, et al. Duplex ultrasound verified by angiography in patients with severe primary and restenosis of internal carotid artery. Ann Vasc Surg. 2006;20(4):478-81. PMID: 16642286.
105. Tu JV, Wang H, Bowyer B, et al. Risk factors for death or stroke after carotid endarterectomy: observations from the Ontario Carotid Endarterectomy Registry. Stroke. 2003;34(11):2568-73. PMID: 14526040.
106. Ungersbock K, Bocher-Schwarz H, Muller-Forell W, et al. The preoperative assessment of stroke risk in lesions involving the internal carotid artery. Br J Neurosurg. 1995;9(4):477-86. PMID: 7576274.
107. Valentine N, Van de Laar FA, van Driel ML. Adenosine-diphosphate (ADP) receptor antagonists for the prevention of cardiovascular disease in type 2 diabetes mellitus. Cochrane Database Syst Rev: John Wiley & Sons, Ltd; 2012.
108. Vernieri F, Pasqualetti P, Matteis M, et al. Effect of collateral blood flow and cerebral vasomotor reactivity on the outcome of carotid artery occlusion. Stroke. 2001;32(7):1552-8. PMID: 11441200.
109. Vikatmaa P, Mitchell D, Jensen LP, et al. Variation in clinical practice in carotid surgery in nine countries 2005-2010. Lessons from VASCUNET and recommendations for the future of national clinical audit. Eur J Vasc Endovasc Surg. 2012;44(1):11-7. PMID: 22633072.
110. Wardlaw JM, Chappell FM, Stevenson M, et al. Accurate, practical and cost-effective assessment of carotid stenosis in the UK (Structured abstract). Health Technol Assess Database. 2006(3):1.
111. Yates GN, Bergamini TM, George SM Jr, et al. Carotid endarterectomy results from a state vascular society. Kentucky Vascular Surgery Society Study Group. Am J Surg. 1997;173(4):342-4. PMID: 9136793.
112. You Y, Hao Q, Leung T, et al. Detection of the siphon internal carotid artery stenosis: transcranial Doppler versus digital subtraction angiography. J Neuroimaging. 2010;20(3):234-9. PMID: 19889048.
113. Zanchetti A, Crepaldi G, Bond MG, et al. Different effects of antihypertensive regimens based on fosinopril or hydrochlorothiazide with or without lipid lowering by pravastatin on progression of asymptomatic carotid atherosclerosis: principal results of PHYLLIS--a randomized double-blind trial. Stroke. 2004;35(12):2807-12. PMID: 15514192.

Ineligible Screening/Intervention

1. Aldoori MI, Benveniste GL, Baird RN, et al. Asymptomatic carotid murmur: ultrasonic factors influencing outcome. Br J Surg. 1987;74(6):496-9. PMID: 3300839.
2. Allen BT, Anderson CB, Rubin BG, et al. The influence of anesthetic technique on perioperative complications after carotid endarterectomy. J Vasc Surg. 1994;19(5):834-42. PMID: 8170037.

Appendix C. Excluded Studies

3. Al-Mubarak N, Roubin GS, Vitek JJ, et al. Microembolization during carotid stenting with the distal-balloon antiemboli system. Int Angiol. 2002;21(4):344-8.
4. Bornstein NM, Gur AY, Geyer O, et al. Vasomotor reactivity in the ophthalmic artery: different from or similar to intracerebral vessels? Eur J Ultrasound. 2000;11(1):1-6. PMID: 10717507.
5. Can U, Furie KL, Suwanwela N, et al. Transcranial Doppler ultrasound criteria for hemodynamically significant internal carotid artery stenosis based on residual lumen diameter calculated from en bloc endarterectomy specimens. Stroke. 1997;28(10):1966-71. PMID: 9341705.
6. Cantelmo NL, Gordon JK, Hyde C, et al. The significance of early postoperative duplex studies following carotid endarterectomy. Cardiovasc Surg. 1999;7(3):298-302. PMID: 10386746.
7. Debrey SM, Yu H, Lynch JK, et al. Diagnostic accuracy of magnetic resonance angiography for internal carotid artery disease: a systematic review and meta-analysis (Structured abstract). Stroke; 2008 :2237-48.
8. Droste DW, Boehm T, Ritter MA, et al. Benefit of echocontrast-enhanced transcranial arterial color-coded duplex ultrasound. Cerebrovasc Dis. 2005;20(5):332-6. PMID: 16131802.
9. Droste DW, Jurgens R, Nabavi DG, et al. Echocontrast-enhanced ultrasound of extracranial internal carotid artery high-grade stenosis and occlusion. Stroke. 1999;30(11):2302-6. PMID: 10548662.
10. Durham CA, Ehlert BA, Agle SC, et al. Role of statin therapy and angiotensin blockade in patients with asymptomatic moderate carotid artery stenosis. Ann Vasc Surg. 2012;26(3):344-52. PMID: 22285349.
11. Illuminati G, Ricco JB, Greco C, et al. Systematic preoperative coronary angiography and stenting improves postoperative results of carotid endarterectomy in patients with asymptomatic coronary artery disease: a randomised controlled trial. Eur J Vasc Endovasc Surg. 2010;39(2):139-45. PMID: 20005750.
12. Kallmes DF, Omary RA, Dix JE, et al. Specificity of MR angiography as a confirmatory test of carotid artery stenosis (Structured abstract). Am J Neuroradiol. 1996:1501-6.
13. Klotzsch C, Popescu O, Sliwka U, et al. Detection of stenoses in the anterior circulation using frequency-based transcranial color-coded sonography. Ultrasound Med Biol. 2000;26(4):579-84. PMID: 10856620.
14. Kretz B, Abello N, Astruc K, et al. Influence of the contralateral carotid artery on carotid surgery outcome. Ann Vasc Surg. 2012;26(6):766-74. PMID: 22717355.
15. Longstreth WT Jr, Shemanski L, Lefkowitz D, et al. Asymptomatic internal carotid artery stenosis defined by ultrasound and the risk of subsequent stroke in the elderly. The Cardiovascular Health Study. Stroke. 1998;29(11):2371-6.
16. Marcucci G, Accrocca F, Gabrielli R, et al. Complete transposition of carotid bifurcation: can it be an additional risk factor of injury to the cranial nerves during carotid endarterectomy? Interact Cardiovasc Thorac Surg. 2011;13(5):471-4. PMID: 21873365.
17. Moll FL, Eikelboom BC, Vermeulen FE, et al. Risk factors in asymptomatic patients with a carotid bruit. Eur J Vasc Surg. 1987;1(1):33-9. PMID: 3503760.
18. Mracek J, Holeckova I, Chytra I, et al. The impact of general versus local anesthesia on early subclinical cognitive function following carotid endarterectomy evaluated using P3 event-related potentials. Acta Neurochir (Wien). 2012;154(3):433-8. PMID: 22245975.
19. Pedro LM, Pedro MM, Goncalves I, et al. Computer-assisted carotid plaque analysis: characteristics of plaques associated with cerebrovascular symptoms and cerebral infarction. Eur J Vasc Endovasc Surg. 2000;19(2):118-23. PMID: 10727359.
20. Pennekamp CW, Tromp SC, Ackerstaff RG, et al. Prediction of cerebral hyperperfusion after carotid endarterectomy with transcranial Doppler. Eur J Vasc Endovasc Surg. 2012;43(4):371-6. PMID: 22264422.
21. Prati P, Tosetto A, Vanuzzo D, et al. Carotid intima media thickness and plaques can predict the occurrence of ischemic cerebrovascular events. Stroke. 2008;39(9):2470-6. PMID: 18617662.
22. Regina G, Angiletta D, Impedovo G, et al. Dexamethasone minimizes the risk of cranial nerve injury during CEA. J Vasc Surg. 2009;49(1):99-102. PMID: 19028044.
23. Schechter MA, Shortell CK, Scarborough JE. Regional versus general anesthesia for carotid endarterectomy: the American College of Surgeons National Surgical Quality Improvement Program perspective. Surgery. 2012;152(3):309-14. PMID: 22749369.
24. Tang TY, Howarth SP, Miller SR, et al. Comparison of the inflammatory burden of truly asymptomatic carotid atheroma with atherosclerotic plaques contralateral to symptomatic carotid stenosis: an ultra small superparamagnetic iron oxide enhanced magnetic resonance study. J Neurol Neurosurg Psychiatry. 2007;78(12):1337-43. PMID: 17578854.
25. Wessels T, Harrer JU, Stetter S, et al. Three-dimensional assessment of extracranial Doppler sonography in carotid artery stenosis compared with digital subtraction angiography. Stroke. 2004;35(8):1847-51. PMID: 15205489.

Appendix C. Excluded Studies

Ineligible Comparator

1. AbuRahma AF, Robinson P, Holt SM, et al. Perioperative and late stroke rates of carotid endarterectomy contralateral to carotid artery occlusion: results from a randomized trial. Stroke. 2000;31(7):1566-71. PMID: 10884455.
2. Aburahma AF, Thiele SP, Wulu JT Jr. Prospective controlled study of the natural history of asymptomatic 60% to 69% carotid stenosis according to ultrasonic plaque morphology. J Vasc Surg. 2002;36(3):437-42. PMID: 12218962.
3. Arya S, Pipinos II, Garg N, et al. Carotid endarterectomy is superior to carotid angioplasty and stenting for perioperative and long-term results. Vasc Endovascular Surg. 2011;45(6):490-8. PMID: 21646236.
4. Bagaev E, Pichlmaier AM, Bisdas T, et al. Contralateral internal carotid artery occlusion impairs early but not 30-day stroke rate following carotid endarterectomy. Angiology. 2010;61(7):705-10. PMID: 20498141.
5. Ballotta E, Da Giau G, Saladini M, et al. Carotid endarterectomy with patch closure versus carotid eversion endarterectomy and reimplantation: a prospective randomized study. Surgery. 1999;125(3):271-9. PMID: 10076611.
6. Bangalore S, Kumar S, Wetterslev J, et al. Carotid artery stenting vs carotid endarterectomy: meta-analysis and diversity-adjusted trial sequential analysis of randomized trials (Structured abstract). Arch Neurol. 2011:172-84.
7. Belcaro G, Laurora G, Cesarone MR, et al. Ultrasonic classification of carotid plaques causing less than 60% stenosis according to ultrasound morphology and events. J Cardiovasc Surg (Torino). 1993;34(4):287-94. PMID: 8227107.
8. Bergeron P, Becquemin JP, Jausseran JM, et al. Percutaneous stenting of the internal carotid artery: the European CAST I study. Carotid Artery Stent Trial. J Endovasc Surg. 1999;6(2):155-9. PMID: 10473333.
9. Blackshear JL, Cutlip DE, Roubin GS, et al. Myocardial infarction after carotid stenting and endarterectomy: results from the carotid revascularization endarterectomy versus stenting trial. Circulation. 2011;123(22):2571-8. PMID: 21606394.
10. Bond R, Rerkasem K, Naylor AR, et al. Systematic review of randomized controlled trials of patch angioplasty versus primary closure and different types of patch materials during carotid endarterectomy (Brief record). J Vasc Surg; 2004:1126-35.
11. Brahmanandam S, Ding EL, Conte MS, et al. Clinical results of carotid artery stenting compared with carotid endarterectomy. J Vasc Surg. 2008;47(2):343-9. PMID: 18241758.
12. Brightwell RE, Sherwood RA, Athanasiou T, et al. The neurological morbidity of carotid revascularisation: using markers of cellular brain injury to compare CEA and CAS. Eur J Vasc Endovasc Surg. 2007;34(5):552-60. PMID: 17719806.
13. Brooks WH, McClure RR, Jones MR, et al. Carotid angioplasty and stenting versus carotid endarterectomy for treatment of asymptomatic carotid stenosis: a randomized trial in a community hospital. Neurosurgery. 2004;54(2):318-24. PMID: 14744277.
14. Cao P, Giordano G, De Rango P, et al. A randomized study on eversion versus standard carotid endarterectomy: study design and preliminary results: the Everest Trial. J Vasc Surg. 1998;27(4):595-605. PMID: 9576071.
15. Counsell CE, Salinas R, Naylor R, et al. A systematic review of the randomised trials of carotid patch angioplasty in carotid endarterectomy. Eur J Vasc Endovasc Surg. 1997;13(4):345-54. PMID: 9133984.
16. Dardik H, Wolodiger F, Silvestri F, et al. Clinical experience with everted cervical vein as patch material after carotid endarterectomy. J Vasc Surg. 1997;25(3):545-53. PMID: 9081137.
17. De Rango P, Lenti M, Simonte G, et al. No benefit from carotid intervention in fatal stroke prevention for >80-year-old patients. Eur J Vasc Endovasc Surg. 2012;44(3):252-9. PMID: 22819739.
18. De Rango P, Verzini F, Cao P, et al. Carotid revascularization provides similar outcomes in symptomatic and asymptomatic patients with <70 years. Stroke. 2012;43(2).
19. Debing E, Van den Brande P. Chronic renal insufficiency and risk of early mortality in patients undergoing carotid endarterectomy. Ann Vasc Surg. 2006;20(5):609-13. PMID: 16741650.
20. Dorigo W, Pulli R, Pratesi G, et al. Early and long-term results of carotid endarterectomy in diabetic patients. J Vasc Surg. 2011;53(1):44-52. PMID: 21050697.
21. Dumont TM, Rughani AI. National trends in carotid artery revascularization surgery. J Neurosurg. 2012;116(6):1251-7. PMID: 22482791.
22. Economopoulos KP, Sergentanis TN, Tsivgoulis G, et al. Carotid artery stenting versus carotid endarterectomy: a comprehensive meta-analysis of short-term and long-term outcomes (Structured abstract). Stroke. 2011:687-92.

Appendix C. Excluded Studies

23. Erzurum VZ, Littooy FN, Steffen G, et al. Outcome of nonoperative management of asymptomatic high-grade carotid stenosis. J Vasc Surg. 2002;36(4):663-7. PMID: 12368722.
24. Estes JM, Guadagnoli E, Wolf R, et al. The impact of cardiac comorbidity after carotid endarterectomy. J Vasc Surg. 1998;28(4):577-84. PMID: 9786249.
25. Faggioli GL, Ferri M, Gargiulo M, et al. A series of 214 carotid stenting procedures: selection criteria, results and potential predictors of success. Ital J Vasc Endovasc Surg. 2006;13(4):167-72.
26. Felli MM, Alunno A, Castiglione A, et al. CEA versus CAS: short-term and mid-term results. Int Angiol. 2012;31(5):420-6.
27. Fiehler J, Jansen O, Berger J, et al. Differences in complication rates among the centres in the SPACE study. Neuroradiology. 2008:1049-53.
28. Forbes TL. Preliminary results of carotid revascularization endarterectomy vs stenting trial (CREST). J Vasc Surg. 2010;51(5):1300-1. PMID: 20420982.
29. Gasparini D, Piccoli G. Extracranial stenting. Cardiovasc Intervent Radiol. 2011;34:485-6.
30. Gossetti B, Gattuso R, Irace L, et al. Embolism to the brain during carotid stenting and surgery. Acta Chir Belg. 2007;107(2):151-4. PMID: 17515263.
31. Gould DA, Birkmeyer JD. Efficacy versus effectiveness of carotid endarterectomy. Eff Clin Pract. 1999;2(1):30-6. PMID: 10346551.
32. Gray WA, Hopkins LN, Yadav S, et al. Protected carotid stenting in high-surgical-risk patients: the ARCHeR results. J Vasc Surg. 2006;44(2):258-68.
33. Gurm HS, Yadav JS, Fayad P, et al. Long-term results of carotid stenting versus endarterectomy in high-risk patients. N Engl J Med. 2008;358(15):1572-9. PMID: 18403765.
34. Handa N, Matsumoto M, Maeda H, et al. Ischemic stroke events and carotid atherosclerosis. Results of the Osaka Follow-up Study for Ultrasonographic Assessment of Carotid Atherosclerosis (the OSACA Study). Stroke. 1995;26(10):1781-6. PMID: 7570725.
35. Holloway RG Jr, Witter DM Jr, Mushlin AI, et al. Carotid endarterectomy trends in the patterns and outcomes of care at academic medical centers, 1990 through 1995. Arch Neurol. 1998;55(1):25-32. PMID: 9443708.
36. Howard VJ, Lutsep HL, Mackey A, et al. Influence of sex on outcomes of stenting versus endarterectomy: a subgroup analysis of the Carotid Revascularization Endarterectomy versus Stenting Trial (CREST). Lancet Neurol. 2011;10(6):530-7. PMID: 21550314.
37. Jackson RS, Sidawy AN, Amdur RL, et al. Obesity is an independent risk factor for death and cardiac complications after carotid endarterectomy. J Am Coll Surg. 2012;214(2):148-55. PMID: 22192895.
38. Jeng JS, Liu HM, Tu YK. Carotid angioplasty with or without stenting versus carotid endarterectomy for carotid artery stenosis: a meta-analysis (Structured abstract). J Neurol Sci. 2008:40-7.
39. Jordan WD Jr, Voellinger DC, Fisher WS, et al. A comparison of carotid angioplasty with stenting versus endarterectomy with regional anesthesia. J Vasc Surg. 1998;28(3):397-402. PMID: 9737448.
40. Kakkos SK, Nicolaides AN, Griffin M, et al. Factors associated with mortality in patients with asymptomatic carotid stenosis: results from the ACSRS study. Int Angiol. 2005;24(3):221-30.
41. Kanter MC, Tegeler CH, Pearce LA, et al. Carotid stenosis in patients with atrial fibrillation. Prevalence, risk factors, and relationship to stroke in the Stroke Prevention in Atrial Fibrillation Study. Arch Intern Med. 1994;154(12):1372-7. PMID: 8002689.
42. Kapral MK, Wang H, Austin PC, et al. Sex differences in carotid endarterectomy outcomes: results from the Ontario Carotid Endarterectomy Registry. Stroke. 2003;34(5):1120-5. PMID: 12690225.
43. Kasirajan K, Matteson B, Marek JM, et al. Comparison of nonneurological events in high-risk patients treated by carotid angioplasty versus endarterectomy. Am J Surg. 2003;185(4):301-4. PMID: 12657378.
44. Kastrup A, Groschel K, Nagele T, et al. Effects of age and symptom status on silent ischemic lesions after carotid stenting with and without the use of distal filter devices. Am J Neuroradiol. 2008;29(3):608-12.
45. Kastrup A, Schulz JB, Raygrotzki S, et al. Comparison of angioplasty and stenting with cerebral protection versus endarterectomy for treatment of internal carotid artery stenosis in elderly patients. J Vasc Surg. 2004;40(5):945-51. PMID: 15557909.
46. Kazmers AE. Caroltid surgery in octogenarians in Veterans Affairs medical centers. J Surg Res. 1999;81.
47. Khatri R, Chaudhry SA, Vazquez G, et al. Age differential between outcomes of carotid angioplasty and stent placement and carotid endarterectomy in general practice. J Vasc Surg. 2012;55(1):72-8. PMID: 22070935.
48. Lanska DJ, Kryscio RJ. In-hospital mortality following carotid endarterectomy. Neurology. 1998;51(2):440-7. PMID: 9710016.
49. Liu Z, Shi Z, Wang Y, et al. Carotid artery stenting versus carotid endarterectomy: systematic review and meta-analysis (Structured abstract). World J Surg. 2009:586-96.

Appendix C. Excluded Studies

50. Luebke T, Aleksic M, Brunkwall J. Meta-analysis of randomized trials comparing carotid endarterectomy and endovascular treatment (Structured abstract). Eur J Vasc Endovasc Surg. 2007:470-9.

51. Madani A, Beletsky V, Tamayo A, et al. High-risk asymptomatic carotid stenosis: ulceration on 3D ultrasound vs TCD microemboli. Neurology. 2011;77(8):744-50. PMID: 21849642.

52. Magnan PE, Caus T, Branchereau A, et al. Internal carotid artery surgery: ten-year results. Ann Vasc Surg. 1993;7(6):521-9. PMID: 8123454.

53. Mantese VA, Timaran CH, Chiu D, et al. The Carotid Revascularization Endarterectomy versus Stenting Trial (CREST): stenting versus carotid endarterectomy for carotid disease. Stroke. 2010;41(10 Suppl):S31-4. PMID: 20876500.

54. Mathiesen EB, Johnsen SH, Wilsgaard T, et al. Carotid plaque area and intima-media thickness in prediction of first-ever ischemic stroke: a 10-year follow-up of 6584 men and women: the Tromso Study. Stroke. 2011;42(4):972-8. PMID: 21311059.

55. Mattos MA, Barkmeier LD, Hodgson KJ, et al. Internal carotid artery occlusion: operative risks and long-term stroke rates after contralateral carotid endarterectomy. Surgery. 1992;112(4):670-9. PMID: 1411937.

56. Maxwell JG, Rutledge R, Covington DL, et al. A statewide, hospital-based analysis of frequency and outcomes in carotid endarterectomy. Am J Surg. 1997;174(6):655-60. PMID: 9409592.

57. Meier P, Knapp G, Tamhane U, et al. Short term and intermediate term comparison of endarterectomy versus stenting for carotid artery stenosis: systematic review and meta-analysis of randomised controlled clinical trials (Structured abstract). BMJ; 2010.

58. Miller MT, Comerota AJ, Tzilinis A, et al. Carotid endarterectomy in octogenarians: does increased age indicate "high risk?". J Vasc Surg. 2005;41(2):231-7. PMID: 15768004.

59. Montauban van Swijndregt AD, Elbers HR, Moll FL, et al. Cerebral ischemic disease and morphometric analyses of carotid plaques. Ann Vasc Surg. 1999;13(5):468-74. PMID: 10466989.

60. Mostaza JM, Gonzalez-Juanatey JR, Castillo J, et al. Prevalence of carotid stenosis and silent myocardial ischemia in asymptomatic subjects with a low ankle-brachial index. J Vasc Surg. 2009;49(1):104-8. PMID: 18829225.

61. Murad MH, Flynn DN, Elamin MB, et al. Endarterectomy vs stenting for carotid artery stenosis: a systematic review and meta-analysis (Structured abstract). J Vasc Surg. 2008:487-93.

62. Murad MH, Shahrour A, Shah ND, et al. A systematic review and meta-analysis of randomized trials of carotid endarterectomy vs stenting (Structured abstract). J Vasc Surg. 2011:792-7.

63. Nonent M, Serfaty JM, Nighoghossian N, et al. Concordance rate differences of 3 noninvasive imaging techniques to measure carotid stenosis in clinical routine practice: results of the CARMEDAS multicenter study. Stroke. 2004;35(3):682-6. PMID: 14764932.

64. Parlani G, De Rango P, Cieri E, et al. Diabetes is not a predictor of outcome for carotid revascularization with stenting as it may be for carotid endarterectomy. J Vasc Surg. 2012;55(1):79-89. PMID: 22056251.

65. Pemberton M, Reid A, London NJ, et al. Carotid endarterectomy is safe in selected elderly patients. Br J Surg. 1998;85(4):507. PMID: 9607533.

66. Perler BA, Dardik A, Burleyson GP, et al. Influence of age and hospital volume on the results of carotid endarterectomy: a statewide analysis of 9918 cases. J Vasc Surg. 1998;27(1):25-31. PMID: 9474079.

67. Pinkerton JJ, Gholkar VR. Should patient age be a consideration in carotid endarterectomy. J Vasc Surg. 1990;11(5).

68. Plecha EJ, King TA, Pitluk HC, et al. Risk assessment in patients undergoing carotid endarterectomy. Cardiovasc Surg. 1993;1(1):30-2. PMID: 8075992.

69. Qureshi AI, Kirmani JF, Divani AA, et al. Carotid angioplasty with or without stent placement versus carotid endarterectomy for treatment of carotid stenosis: a meta-analysis (Structured abstract). Neurosurgery. 2005:1171-9.

70. Rerkasem K, Rothwell PM. Systematic review of randomized controlled trials of patch angioplasty versus primary closure during carotid endarterectomy (Brief record). Stroke. 2010:e55-6.

71. Rigdon EE, Monajjem N, Rhodes RS. Is carotid endarterectomy justified in patients with severe chronic renal insufficiency? Ann Vasc Surg. 1997;11(2):115-9. PMID: 9181764.

72. Riles TS, Lee V, Cheever D, et al. Clinical course of asymptomatic patients with carotid duplex scan end diastolic velocities of 100 to 124 centimeters per second. J Vasc Surg. 2010;52(4):914-9. PMID: 20630689.

73. Rothwell PM, Slattery J, Warlow CP. A systematic comparison of the risks of stroke and death due to carotid endarterectomy for symptomatic and asymptomatic stenosis (Structured abstract). Stroke. 1996:266-9.

Appendix C. Excluded Studies

74. Rudarakanchana N, Dialynas M, Halliday A. Asymptomatic Carotid Surgery Trial-2 (ACST-2): rationale for a randomised clinical trial comparing carotid endarterectomy with carotid artery stenting in patients with asymptomatic carotid artery stenosis. Eur J Vasc Endovasc Surg. 2009;38(2):239-42.
75. Saba L, Sanfilippo R, Montisci R, et al. Correlation between US-PSV and MDCTA in the quantification of carotid artery stenosis. Eur J Radiol. 2010;74(1):99-103. PMID: 19246169.
76. Schneider EB, Black JH 3rd, Hambridge HL, et al. The impact of race and ethnicity on the outcome of carotid interventions in the United States. J Surg Res. 2012;177(1):172-7. PMID: 22459294.
77. Sheffet AJ, Roubin G, Howard G, et al. Design of the Carotid Revascularization Endarterectomy vs. Stenting Trial (CREST). Int J Stroke. 2010;5(1):40-6.
78. Siebler M, Nachtmann A, Sitzer M, et al. Cerebral microembolism and the risk of ischemia in asymptomatic high-grade internal carotid artery stenosis. Stroke. 1995;26(11):2184-6. PMID: 7482670.
79. Stanziale SF, Marone LK, Boules TN, et al. Carotid artery stenting in octogenarians is associated with increased adverse outcomes. J Vasc Surg. 2006;43(2):297-304. PMID: 16476605.
80. Steinke W, Meairs S, Ries S, et al. Sonographic assessment of carotid artery stenosis. Comparison of power Doppler imaging and color Doppler flow imaging. Stroke. 1996;27(1):91-4. PMID: 8553411.
81. Stukenborg GJ. Comparison of carotid endarterectomy outcomes from randomized controlled trials and Medicare administrative databases. Arch Neurol. 1997;54(7):826-32. PMID: 9236570.
82. Theiss W, Hermanek P, Mathias K, et al. Pro-CAS: a prospective registry of carotid angioplasty and stenting. Stroke. 2004;35(9):2134-9. PMID: 15232119.
83. Touze E, Trinquart L, Chatellier G, et al. Systematic review of the perioperative risks of stroke or death after carotid angioplasty and stenting (Structured abstract). Stroke. 2009:e683-93.
84. Usman AA, Tang GL, Eskandari MK. Metaanalysis of procedural stroke and death among octogenarians: carotid stenting versus carotid endarterectomy. J Am Coll Surg. 2009;208(6):1124-31. PMID: 19476901.
85. Warlow CP, Bodenham AR, Colam B, et al. General anaesthesia versus local anaesthesia for carotid surgery (GALA): a multicentre, randomised controlled trial. Lancet. 2008;372(9656):2132-42.
86. White RA, Sicard GA, Zwolak RM, et al. Society of vascular surgery vascular registry comparison of carotid artery stenting outcomes for atherosclerotic vs nonatherosclerotic carotid artery disease. J Vasc Surg. 2010;51(5):1116-23. PMID: 20347551.
87. Wiesmann M, Schopf V, Jansen O, et al. Stent-protected angioplasty versus carotid endarterectomy in patients with carotid artery stenosis: meta-analysis of randomized trial data (Structured abstract). Eur Radiol. 2008:2956-66.
88. Yavin D, Roberts DJ, Tso M, et al. Carotid endarterectomy versus stenting: a meta-analysis of randomized trials (Structured abstract). Can J Neurol Sci. 2011:230-5.
89. Yeh RW, Kennedy K, Spertus JA, et al. Do postmarketing surveillance studies represent real-world populations? A comparison of patient characteristics and outcomes after carotid artery stenting. Circulation. 2011;123(13):1384-90. PMID: 21422383.
90. Zahn R, Hochadel M, Grau A, et al. Stent-supported angioplasty versus endarterectomy for carotid artery stenosis: evidence from current randomized trials (Structured abstract). Z Kardiol. 2005:836-43.

Ineligible Outcome

1. Adachi T, Takagi M, Hoshino H, et al. Effect of extracranial carotid artery stenosis and other risk factors for stroke on periventricular hyperintensity. Stroke. 1997;28(11):2174-9. PMID: 9368560.
2. Beijers HJ, Henry RM, Bravenboer B, et al. Metabolic syndrome in nondiabetic individuals associated with maladaptive carotid remodeling: the Hoorn Study. Am J Hypertens. 2011;24(4):429-36. PMID: 21212746.
3. Bicknell CD, Cowling MG, Clark MW, et al. Carotid angioplasty in a pulsatile flow model: factors affecting embolic potential. Eur J Vasc Endovasc Surg. 2003;26(1):22-31. PMID: 12819644.
4. Cohen SN, Hobson RW 2nd, Weiss DG, et al. Death associated with asymptomatic carotid artery stenosis: long-term clinical evaluation. VA Cooperative Study 167 Group. J Vasc Surg. 1993;18(6):1002-9. PMID: 8264028.
5. Comerota AJ, Salles-Cunha SX, Daoud Y, et al. Gender differences in blood velocities across carotid stenoses. J Vasc Surg. 2004;40(5):939-44. PMID: 15557908.
6. Cote R, Battista RN, Abrahamowicz M, et al. Lack of effect of aspirin in asymptomatic patients with carotid bruits and substantial carotid narrowing. The Asymptomatic Cervical Bruit Study Group. Ann Intern Med. 1995;123(9):649-55. PMID: 7574219.

Appendix C. Excluded Studies

7. Cuspidi C, Meani S, Valerio C, et al. Carotid atherosclerosis and cardiovascular risk stratification: role and cost-effectiveness of echo-Doppler examination in untreated essential hypertensives. Blood Press. 2006;15(6):333-9. PMID: 17472023.
8. Deriu GP, Milite D, Damiani N, et al. Carotid endarterectomy without angiography: a prospective randomised pilot study. Eur J Vasc Endovasc Surg. 2000;20(3):250-3. PMID: 10986023.
9. Feasby TE, Quan H, Ghali WA. Provincial carotid endarterectomy outcomes. Can J Neurol Sci. 2002;29(4):333-6. PMID: 12463488.
10. Fried LP, Borhani NO, Enright P, et al. The Cardiovascular Health Study: design and rationale. Ann Epidemiol. 1991;1(3):263-76. PMID: 1669507.
11. Hartmann A, Mast H, Thompson JL, et al. Transcranial Doppler waveform blunting in severe extracranial carotid artery stenosis. Cerebrovasc Dis. 2000;10(1):33-8. PMID: 10629344.
12. Heliopoulos J, Vadikolias K, Piperidou C, et al. Detection of carotid artery plaque ulceration using 3-dimensional ultrasound. J Neuroimaging. 2011;21(2):126-31.
13. Heyman A, Wilkinson WE, Heyden S, et al. Risk of stroke in asymptomatic persons with cervical arterial bruits: a population study in Evans County, Georgia. N Engl J Med. 1980;302(15):838-41. PMID: 7360161.
14. Horn J, Naylor AR, Laman DM, et al. Identification of patients at risk for ischaemic cerebral complications after carotid endarterectomy with TCD monitoring. Eur J Vasc Endovasc Surg. 2005;30(3):270-4. PMID: 15963744.
15. Kardoulas DG, Katsamouris AN, Gallis PT, et al. Ultrasonographic and histologic characteristics of symptom-free and symptomatic carotid plaque. Cardiovasc Surg. 1996;4(5):580-90. PMID: 8909814.
16. Kim SH, Kim YM, Cho MA, et al. Echogenic carotid artery plaques are associated with vertebral fractures in postmenopausal women with low bone mass. Calcif Tissue Int. 2008;82(6):411-7. PMID: 18496724.
17. Lal BK, Brott TG. The Carotid Revascularization Endarterectomy vs. Stenting Trial completes randomization: lessons learned and anticipated results. J Vasc Surg. 2009;50(5):1224-31. PMID: 19878793.
18. Lind L, Andersson J, Hansen T, et al. Atherosclerosis measured by whole body magnetic resonance angiography and carotid artery ultrasound is related to arterial compliance, but not to endothelium-dependent vasodilation. The Prospective Investigation of the Vasculature in Uppsala Seniors (PIVUS) study. Clin Physiol Funct Imaging. 2009;29(5):321-9.
19. Loncar R, Muller BT, Zotz RB, et al. The screening power of methylenetetrahydrofolate reductase C677T polymorphism versus plasma homocysteine concentration in patients with stenosis of the internal carotid artery. Thromb J. 2006;4:16. PMID: 16999862.
20. Mackinnon AD, Aaslid R, Markus HS. Ambulatory transcranial Doppler cerebral embolic signal detection in symptomatic and asymptomatic carotid stenosis. Stroke. 2005;36(8):1726-30. PMID: 16040594.
21. Markus H. The Asymptomatic Carotid Emboli Study: study design and baseline results. Int J Stroke. 2009;4(5):398-405.
22. Newman AB, Naydeck BL, Ives DG, et al. Coronary artery calcium, carotid artery wall thickness, and cardiovascular disease outcomes in adults 70 to 99 years old. Am J Cardiol. 2008;101(2):186-92.
23. Rajeswaran D, Saunder A, Raymond S. Post-operative risk factor control following internal carotid artery intervention. ANZ J Surg. 2011;81(11):817-21. PMID: 22295407.
24. Reiff T, Stingele R, Eckstein HH, et al. Stent-protected angioplasty in asymptomatic carotid artery stenosis vs. endarterectomy: SPACE2--a three-arm randomised-controlled clinical trial. Int J Stroke. 2009;4(4):294-9. PMID: 19689759.
25. Robless P, Emson M, Thomas D, et al. Are we detecting and operating on high risk patients in the asymptomatic carotid surgery trial? The Asymptomatic Carotid Surgery Trial Collaborators. Eur J Vasc Endovasc Surg. 1998;16(1):59-64.
26. Takahashi W, Ohnuki T, Honma K, et al. The significance of multiple risk factors for early carotid atherosclerosis in Japanese subjects. Intern Med. 2007;46(20):1679-84.
27. Tell GS, Fried LP, Hermanson B, et al. Recruitment of adults 65 years and older as participants in the Cardiovascular Health Study. Ann Epidemiol. 1993;3(4):358-66. PMID: 8275211.
28. Voeks JH, Howard G, Roubin GS, et al. Age and outcomes after carotid stenting and endarterectomy: the carotid revascularization endarterectomy versus stenting trial. Stroke. 2011;42(12):3484-90. PMID: 21980205.
29. Wallaert JB, Cronenwett JL, Bertges DJ, et al. Optimal selection of asymptomatic patients for carotid endarterectomy based on predicted 5-year survival. J Vasc Surg. 2013;58(1):112-8. PMID: 23478502.
30. Wiebers DO, Whisnant JP, Sandok BA, et al. Prospective comparison of a cohort with asymptomatic carotid bruit and a population-based cohort without carotid bruit. Stroke. 1990;21(7):984-8. PMID: 2368113.

Appendix C. Excluded Studies

31. Yoshimura S, Kawasaki M, Yamada K, et al. Visualization of internal carotid artery atherosclerotic plaques in symptomatic and asymptomatic patients: a comparison of optical coherence tomography and intravascular ultrasound. AJNR Am J Neuroradiol. 2012;33(2):308-13. PMID: 22051806.

Ineligible Setting

1. Kakkos SK, Sabetai M, Tegos T, et al. Silent embolic infarcts on computed tomography brain scans and risk of ipsilateral hemispheric events in patients with asymptomatic internal carotid artery stenosis. J Vasc Surg. 2009;49(4):902-9. PMID: 19223148.
2. Yurdakul M, Tola M, Cumhur T. B-flow imaging of internal carotid artery stenosis: comparison with power Doppler imaging and digital subtraction angiography. J Clin Ultrasound. 2004;32(5):243-8. PMID: 15124191.

Ineligible Study Design

1. Risk of stroke in the distribution of an asymptomatic carotid artery. The European Carotid Surgery Trialists Collaborative Group. Lancet. 1995;345(8944):209-12. PMID: 7823712.
2. Abbott AL. Medical (nonsurgical) intervention alone is now best for prevention of stroke associated with asymptomatic severe carotid stenosis: results of a systematic review and analysis. Stroke. 2009;40(10):e573-83. PMID: 19696421.
3. Abbott AL, Chambers BR, Stork JL, et al. Embolic signals and prediction of ipsilateral stroke or transient ischemic attack in asymptomatic carotid stenosis: a multicenter prospective cohort study. Stroke. 2005;36(6):1128-33. PMID: 15879327.
4. AbuRahma AF, Metz MJ, Robinson PA. Natural history of ≥60% asymptomatic carotid stenosis in patients with contralateral carotid occlusion. Ann Surg. 2003;238(4):551-61. PMID: 14530726.
5. AbuRahma AF, Srivastava M, Chong B, et al. Impact of chronic renal insufficiency using serum creatinine vs glomerular filtration rate on perioperative clinical outcomes of carotid endarterectomy. J Am Coll Surg. 2013;216(4):525-32. PMID: 23403138.
6. Ackerstaff RG, Vos JA. TCD-detected cerebral embolism in carotid endarterectomy versus angioplasty and stenting of the carotid bifurcation. Acta Chir Belg. 2004;104(1):55-9. PMID: 15053466.
7. Ackerstaff RG. Transcranial Doppler monitoring in angioplasty and stenting of the carotid bifurcation. J Endovasc Ther. 2003;10(4):702-10.
8. Adler Y, Levinger U, Koren A, et al. Relation of nonobstructive aortic valve calcium to carotid arterial atherosclerosis. Am J Cardiol. 2000;86(10):1102-5. PMID: 11074207.
9. Andrawes WF, Bussy C, Belmin J. Prevention of cardiovascular events in elderly people. Drugs Aging. 2005;22(10):859-76. PMID: 16245959.
10. Appleberg M, Cottier D, Crozier J, et al. Carotid endarterectomy for asymptomatic carotid artery stenosis: patients with severe bilateral disease a high risk subgroup. Aust N Z J Surg. 1995;65(3):160-5. PMID: 7887857.
11. Ascher E, Hingorani A, Gunduz Y, et al. Posterior transverse plication technique for treatment of redundant internal carotid artery during endarterectomy. Cardiovasc Surg. 2001;9(1):16-9. PMID: 11137803.
12. Back MR, Rogers GA, Wilson JS, et al. Magnetic resonance angiography minimizes need for arteriography after inadequate carotid duplex ultrasound scanning. J Vasc Surg. 2003;38(3):422-30. PMID: 12947246.
13. Balestrini S, Lupidi F, Balucani C, et al. One-year progression of moderate asymptomatic carotid stenosis predicts the risk of vascular events. Stroke. 2013;44(3):792-4. PMID: 23287778.
14. Ballotta E, Da Giau G, Abbruzzese E, et al. Carotid endarterectomy without angiography: can clinical evaluation and duplex ultrasonographic scanning alone replace traditional arteriography for carotid surgery workup? A prospective study. Surgery. 1999;126(1):20-7.
15. Ballotta E, Meneghetti G, Manara R, et al. Long-term survival and stroke-free survival after eversion carotid endarterectomy for asymptomatic severe carotid stenosis. J Vasc Surg. 2007;46(2):265-70. PMID: 17600662.
16. Bertges DJ, Goodney PP, Zhao Y, et al. The Vascular Study Group of New England Cardiac Risk Index (VSG-CRI) predicts cardiac complications more accurately than the Revised Cardiac Risk Index in vascular surgery patients. J Vasc Surg. 2010;52(3):674-83. PMID: 20570467.
17. Bisdas T, Egorova N, Moskowitz AJ, et al. The impact of gender on in-hospital outcomes after carotid endarterectomy or stenting. Eur J Vasc Endovasc Surg. 2012;44(3):244-50. PMID: 22819738.
18. Bots ML, Breslau PJ, Briet E, et al. Cardiovascular determinants of carotid artery disease. The Rotterdam Elderly Study. Hypertension. 1992;19(6 Pt 2):717-20. PMID: 1592472.

Appendix C. Excluded Studies

19. Boules TN, Proctor MC, Aref A, et al. Carotid endarterectomy remains the standard of care, even in high-risk surgical patients. Ann Surg. 2005;241(2):356-63. PMID: 15650648.
20. Brajovic MD, Markovic N, Loncar G, et al. The influence of various morphologic and hemodynamic carotid plaque characteristics on neurological events onset and deaths. Sci World J. 2009;9:509-21.
21. Bunch CT, Kresowik TF. Can randomized trial outcomes for carotid endarterectomy be achieved in community-wide practice? Semin Vasc Surg. 2004;17(3):209-13. PMID: 15449242.
22. Buszman PP, Szymanski R, Debinski M, et al. Long-term results of cephalad arteries percutanoeus transluminal angioplasty with stent implantation (the CAPTAS registry). Catheter Cardiovasc Interv. 2012;79(4):532-40. PMID: 22311860.
23. Calvillo-King L, Xuan L, Zhang S, et al. Predicting risk of perioperative death and stroke after carotid endarterectomy in asymptomatic patients: derivation and validation of a clinical risk score. Stroke. 2010;41(12):2786-94. PMID: 21051669.
24. Cao P, Giordano G, De Rango P, et al. Computerised tomography findings as a risk factor in carotid endarterectomy: early and late results. Eur J Vasc Endovasc Surg. 1996;12(1):37-45. PMID: 8696895.
25. Cao P, Zannetti S, Giordano G, et al. Cerebral tomographic findings in patients undergoing carotid endarterectomy for asymptomatic carotid stenosis: short-term and long-term implications. J Vasc Surg. 1999;29(6):995-1005. PMID: 10359933.
26. Caracci BF, Zukowski AJ, Hurley JJ, et al. Asymptomatic severe carotid stenosis. J Vasc Surg. 1989;9(2):361-6. PMID: 2645445.
27. Chaves C, Hreib K, Allam G, et al. Patterns of cerebral perfusion in patients with asymptomatic internal carotid artery disease. Cerebrovasc Dis. 2006;22(5-6):396-401. PMID: 16888382.
28. Cinat ME, Casalme C, Wilson SE, et al. Computed tomography angiography validates duplex sonographic evaluation of carotid artery stenosis. Am Surg. 2003;69(10):842-7. PMID: 14570360.
29. Coe DA, Towne JB, Seabrook GR, et al. Duplex morphologic features of the reconstructed carotid artery: changes occurring more than five years after endarterectomy. J Vasc Surg. 1997;25(5):850-6. PMID: 9152312.
30. Dalainas I, Nano G, Bianchi P, et al. Carotid endarterectomy in patients with contralateral carotid artery occlusion. Ann Vasc Surg. 2007;21(1):16-22.
31. Dardik A, Bowman HM, Gordon TA, et al. Impact of race on the outcome of carotid endarterectomy: a population-based analysis of 9,842 recent elective procedures. Ann Surg. 2000;232(5):704-9. PMID: 11066143.
32. de Donato G, Setacci C, Deloose K, et al. Long-term results of carotid artery stenting. J Vasc Surg. 2008;48(6):1431-40. PMID: 18848755.
33. Debing E, Aerden D, Van den Brande P. Diabetes mellitus is a predictor for early adverse outcome after carotid endarterectomy. Vasc Endovascular Surg. 2011;45(1):28-32. PMID: 21156716.
34. Debing E, Van den Brande P. Carotid endarterectomy in the elderly: are the patient characteristics, the early outcome, and the predictors the same as those in younger patients? Surg Neurol. 2007;67(5):467-71. PMID: 17445605.
35. den Hartog AG, Achterberg S, Moll FL, et al. Asymptomatic carotid artery stenosis and the risk of ischemic stroke according to subtype in patients with clinical manifest arterial disease. Stroke. 2013;44(4):1002-7. PMID: 23404720.
36. Duschek N, Ghai S, Sejkic F, et al. Homocysteine improves risk stratification in patients undergoing endarterectomy for asymptomatic internal carotid artery stenosis. Stroke. 2013;44(8):2311-4. PMID: 23760214.
37. Eldrup N, Gronholdt ML, Sillesen H, et al. Elevated matrix metalloproteinase-9 associated with stroke or cardiovascular death in patients with carotid stenosis. Circulation. 2006;114(17):1847-54. PMID: 17030690.
38. Fine-Edelstein JS, Wolf PA, O'Leary DH, et al. Precursors of extracranial carotid atherosclerosis in the Framingham study. Neurology. 1994;44(6):1046-50.
39. Finocchi C, Gandolfo C, Carissimi T, et al. Role of transcranial Doppler and stump pressure during carotid endarterectomy. Stroke. 1997;28(12):2448-52. PMID: 9412630.
40. Flanigan DP, Flanigan ME, Dorne AL, et al. Long-term results of 442 consecutive, standardized carotid endarterectomy procedures in standard-risk and high-risk patients. J Vasc Surg. 2007;46(5):876-82. PMID: 17980273.
41. Folkersen L, Persson J, Ekstrand J, et al. Prediction of ischemic events on the basis of transcriptomic and genomic profiling in patients undergoing carotid endarterectomy. Mol Med. 2012;18:669-75. PMID: 22371308.
42. Frawley JE, Hicks RG, Woodforth IJ. Risk factors for peri-operative stroke complicating carotid endarterectomy: selective analysis of a prospective audit of 1000 consecutive operations. Aust N Z J Surg. 2000;70(1):52-6. PMID: 10696944.

Appendix C. Excluded Studies

43. Furst H, Hartl WH, Haberl R, et al. Silent cerebral infarction: risk factor for stroke complicating carotid endarterectomy. World J Surg. 2001;25(8):969-74. PMID: 11571977.
44. Garvey L, Makaroun MS, Muluk VS, et al. Etiologic factors in progression of carotid stenosis: a 10-year study in 905 patients. J Vasc Surg. 2000;31(1 Pt 1):31-8. PMID: 10642706.
45. Goldstein LB, Samsa GP, Matchar DB, et al. Multicenter review of preoperative risk factors for endarterectomy for asymptomatic carotid artery stenosis. Stroke. 1998;29(4):750-3. PMID: 9550506.
46. Goliasch G, Schillinger M, Mayer FJ, et al. Usefulness of hemoglobin level to predict long-term mortality in patients with asymptomatic carotid narrowing by ultrasonography. Am J Cardiol. 2012;110(11):1699-703.
47. Greco G, Egorova NN, Moskowitz AJ, et al. A model for predicting the risk of carotid artery disease. Ann Surg. 2013;257(6):1168-73. PMID: 23333880.
48. Griewing B, Morgenstern C, Driesner F, et al. Cerebrovascular disease assessed by color-flow and power Doppler ultrasonography. Comparison with digital subtraction angiography in internal carotid artery stenosis. Stroke. 1996;27(1):95-100. PMID: 8553412.
49. Grizzell BE, Ammar AD, Helmer SD. Carotid stenosis: change of treatment plan based on repeat duplex ultrasonography. Am J Surg. 2012;203(2):121-6. PMID: 21784407.
50. Gronholdt ML, Nordestgaard BG, Schroeder TV, et al. Ultrasonic echolucent carotid plaques predict future strokes. Circulation. 2001;104(1):68-73. PMID: 11435340.
51. Groschel K, Ernemann U, Riecker A, et al. Incidence and risk factors for medical complications after carotid artery stenting. J Vasc Surg. 2005;42(6):1101-6. PMID: 16376198.
52. Halliday A, Bulbulia R, Gray W, et al. Status update and interim results from the asymptomatic carotid surgery trial-2 (ACST-2). Eur J Vasc Endovasc Surg. 2013;46(5):510-8. PMID: 24051108.
53. Hamdan AD, Pomposelli FB Jr, Gibbons GW, et al. Renal insufficiency and altered postoperative risk in carotid endarterectomy. J Vasc Surg. 1999;29(6):1006-11. PMID: 10359934.
54. Harthun NL, Stukenborg GJ. Atrial fibrillation is associated with increased risk of perioperative stroke and death from carotid endarterectomy. J Vasc Surg. 2010;51(2):330-6. PMID: 19879714.
55. Hawkins BM, Kennedy KF, Giri J, et al. Pre-procedural risk quantification for carotid stenting using the CAS score: a report from the NCDR CARE Registry. J Am Coll Cardiol. 2012;60(17):1617-22. PMID: 22999733.
56. Heyer EJ, Mergeche JL, Bruce SS, et al. Statins reduce neurologic injury in asymptomatic carotid endarterectomy patients. Stroke. 2013;44(4):1150-2. PMID: 23404722.
57. Hobson IR, Krupski WC, Weiss DG, et al. Influence of aspirin in the management of asymptomatic carotid artery stenosis. J Vasc Surg. 1993;17(2):257-65.
58. Hobson RW 2nd, Howard VJ, Roubin GS, et al. Carotid artery stenting is associated with increased complications in octogenarians: 30-day stroke and death rates in the CREST lead-in phase. J Vasc Surg. 2004;40(6):1106-11. PMID: 15622363.
59. Hoke M, Schillinger M, Dick P, et al. Polymorphism of the palladin gene and cardiovascular outcome in patients with atherosclerosis. Eur J Clin Invest. 2011;41(4):365-71. PMID: 21054356.
60. Hoke M, Speidl W, Schillinger M, et al. Polymorphism of the complement 5 gene and cardiovascular outcome in patients with atherosclerosis. Eur J Clin Invest. 2012;42(9):921-6. PMID: 22452399.
61. Iihara K, Murao K, Sakai N, et al. Outcome of carotid endarterectomy and stent insertion based on grading of carotid endarterectomy risk: a 7-year prospective study. J Neurosurg. 2006;105(4):546-54. PMID: 17044557.
62. Jansen C, Sprengers AM, Moll FL, et al. Prediction of intracerebral haemorrhage after carotid endarterectomy by clinical criteria and intraoperative transcranial Doppler monitoring. Eur J Vasc Surg. 1994;8(3):303-8. PMID: 7912206.
63. Jaroslav P, Christian R, Stefan O, et al. Evaluation of serum biomarkers for patients at increased risk of stroke. Int J Vasc Med. 2012;2012.
64. Joakimsen O, Bonaa KH, Mathiesen EB, et al. Prediction of mortality by ultrasound screening of a general population for carotid stenosis: the Tromso Study. Stroke. 2000;31(8):1871-6. PMID: 10926949.
65. Kakkos SK, Griffin MB, Nicolaides AN, et al. The size of juxtaluminal hypoechoic area in ultrasound images of asymptomatic carotid plaques predicts the occurrence of stroke. J Vasc Surg. 2013;57(3):609-18. PMID: 23337294.
66. Kasper GC, Lohr JM, Welling RE. Clinical benefit of carotid endarterectomy based on duplex ultrasonography. Vasc Endovascular Surg. 2003;37(5):323-7. PMID: 14528377.
67. Kastrup A, Groschel K, Schulz JB, et al. Clinical predictors of transient ischemic attack, stroke, or death within 30 days of carotid angioplasty and stenting. Stroke. 2005;36(4):787-91. PMID: 15705938.
68. Kawahito S, Kitahata H, Tanaka K, et al. Risk factors for perioperative myocardial ischemia in carotid artery endarterectomy. J Cardiothorac Vasc Anesth. 2004;18(3):288-92. PMID: 15232807.

Appendix C. Excluded Studies

69. King A, Serena J, Bornstein NM, et al. Does impaired cerebrovascular reactivity predict stroke risk in asymptomatic carotid stenosis? A prospective substudy of the asymptomatic carotid emboli study. Stroke. 2011;42(6):1550-5. PMID: 21527764.

70. King A, Shipley M, Markus H. Optimizing protocols for risk prediction in asymptomatic carotid stenosis using embolic signal detection: the Asymptomatic Carotid Emboli Study. Stroke. 2011;42(10):2819-24. PMID: 21852607.

71. Kitamura A, Iso H, Imano H, et al. Carotid intima-media thickness and plaque characteristics as a risk factor for stroke in Japanese elderly men. Stroke. 2004;35(12):2788-94. PMID: 15528460.

72. Krapf H, Nagele T, Kastrup A, et al. Risk factors for periprocedural complications in carotid artery stenting without filter protection: a serial diffusion-weighted MRI study. J Neurol. 2006;253(3):364-71.

73. Lacroix P, Aboyans V, Criqui MH, et al. Type-2 diabetes and carotid stenosis: a proposal for a screening strategy in asymptomatic patients. Vasc Med. 2006;11(2):93-9. PMID: 16886839.

74. Lam TD, Lammers S, Munoz C, et al. Diabetes, intracranial stenosis and microemboli in asymptomatic carotid stenosis. Can J Neurol Sci. 2013;40(2):177-81. PMID: 23419564.

75. Macchi C, Catini C, Giannelli F. The original caliber of the carotid artery as a possible risk factor for complications of atherosclerosis. Ital J Anat Embryol. 1993;98(4):259-68. PMID: 8018017.

76. Mannami T, Baba S, Ogata J. Strong and significant relationships between aggregation of major coronary risk factors and the acceleration of carotid atherosclerosis in the general population of a Japanese City: the Suita Study. Arch Intern Med. 2000;160(15):2297-303.

77. Mansour MA, Littooy FN, Watson WC, et al. Outcome of moderate carotid artery stenosis in patients who are asymptomatic. J Vasc Surg. 1999;29(2):217-25. PMID: 9950980.

78. Marek J, Mills JL, Harvich J, et al. Utility of routine carotid duplex screening in patients who have claudication. J Vasc Surg. 1996;24(4):572-7. PMID: 8911405.

79. Markus HS, King A, Shipley M, et al. Asymptomatic embolisation for prediction of stroke in the Asymptomatic Carotid Emboli Study (ACES): a prospective observational study. Lancet Neurol. 2010;9(7):663-71. PMID: 20554250.

80. Matsumura JS, Gray W, Chaturvedi S, et al. Results of carotid artery stenting with distal embolic protection with improved systems: Protected Carotid Artery Stenting in Patients at High Risk for Carotid Endarterectomy (PROTECT) trial. J Vasc Surg. 2012;55(4):968-76. PMID: 22236885.

81. McCollum PT, da Silva A, Ridler BD, et al. Carotid endarterectomy in the U.K. and Ireland: audit of 30-day outcome. The Audit Committee for the Vascular Surgical Society. Eur J Vasc Endovasc Surg. 1997;14(5):386-91. PMID: 9413380.

82. McCrory DC, Goldstein LB, Samsa GP, et al. Predicting complications of carotid endarterectomy. Stroke. 1993;24(9):1285-91. PMID: 8362419.

83. McDonald RJ, Cloft HJ, Kallmes DF. Intracranial hemorrhage is much more common after carotid stenting than after endarterectomy: evidence from the National Inpatient Sample. Stroke. 2011;42(10):2782-7. PMID: 21836092.

84. Micieli G, Cavallini A, Bosone D, et al. Carotid artery atherosclerosis and risk factors for stroke in a selected population of asymptomatic men. Funct Neurol. 1998;13(1):27-35.

85. Mineva PP, Manchev IC, Hadjiev DI. Prevalence and outcome of asymptomatic carotid stenosis: a population-based ultrasonographic study. Eur J Neurol. 2002;9(4):383-8. PMID: 12099923.

86. Mohan IV, Thomas SD. Do patients with asymptomatic carotid stenoses still benefit from surgical intervention? ANZ J Surg. 2011;81(4):211-3. PMID: 21418460.

87. Molloy J, Markus HS. Asymptomatic embolization predicts stroke and TIA risk in patients with carotid artery stenosis. Stroke. 1999;30(7):1440-3. PMID: 10390320.

88. Momjian-Mayor I, Kuzmanovic I, Momjian S, et al. Accuracy of a novel risk index combining degree of stenosis of the carotid artery and plaque surface echogenicity. Stroke. 2012;43(5):1260-5. PMID: 22403049.

89. Moneta GL, Taylor DC, Zierler RE, et al. Asymptomatic high-grade internal carotid artery stenosis: is stratification according to risk factors or duplex spectral analysis possible? J Vasc Surg. 1989;10(5):475-82. PMID: 2681840.

90. Mono ML, Karameshev A, Slotboom J, et al. Plaque characteristics of asymptomatic carotid stenosis and risk of stroke. Cerebrovasc Dis. 2012;34(5-6):343-50.

91. Morales MM, Anacleto A, Buchdid MA, et al. Morphological and hemodynamic patterns of carotid stenosis treated by endarterectomy with patch closure versus stenting: a duplex ultrasound study. Clinics (Sao Paulo). 2010;65(12):1315-23. PMID: 21340221.

Appendix C. Excluded Studies

92. Mozes G, Sullivan TM, Torres-Russotto DR, et al. Carotid endarterectomy in SAPPHIRE-eligible high-risk patients: implications for selecting patients for carotid angioplasty and stenting. J Vasc Surg. 2004;39(5):958-65. PMID: 15111844.

93. Mullenix PS, Martin MJ, Steele SR, et al. Rapid high-volume population screening for three major risk factors of future stroke: phase I results. Vasc Endovasc Surg. 2006;40(3):177-87.

94. Muller M, Reiche W, Langenscheidt P, et al. Ischemia after carotid endarterectomy: comparison between transcranial Doppler sonography and diffusion-weighted MR imaging. AJNR Am J Neuroradiol. 2000;21(1):47-54. PMID: 10669224.

95. Nicolaides AN, Kakkos SK, Kyriacou E, et al. Asymptomatic internal carotid artery stenosis and cerebrovascular risk stratification. J Vasc Surg. 2010;52(6):1486-96. PMID: 21146746.

96. Nolan BW, De Martino RR, Goodney PP, et al. Comparison of carotid endarterectomy and stenting in real world practice using a regional quality improvement registry. J Vasc Surg. 2012;56(4):990-6. PMID: 22579135.

97. Papalambros E, Georgopoulos S, Sigala F, et al. Changes in circulating levels of vascular endothelial growth factor and vascular endothelial growth factor receptor-2 after carotid endarterectomy. Int J Mol Med. 2004;14(1):133-6. PMID: 15202028.

98. Park BD, Divinagracia T, Madej O, et al. Predictors of clinically significant postprocedural hypotension after carotid endarterectomy and carotid angioplasty with stenting. J Vasc Surg. 2009;50(3):526-33. PMID: 19700091.

99. Persson J, Folkersen L, Ekstrand J, et al. High plasma adiponectin concentration is associated with all-cause mortality in patients with carotid atherosclerosis. Atherosclerosis. 2012;225(2):491-6.

100. Pistolese GR, Ippoliti A, Appolloni A, et al. Cerebral haemodynamics during carotid cross-clamping. Eur J Vasc Surg. 1993;7(Suppl A):33-8. PMID: 8458444.

101. Pitoulias GA, Tachtsi MD, Tsiaousis PZ, et al. Hyperhomocysteinemia and hypercoagulable state in carotid plaque evolution. Novel risk factors or coincidental risk predictors? Int Angiol. 2007;26(3):270-8. PMID: 17622211.

102. Prati P, Tosetto A, Casaroli M, et al. Carotid plaque morphology improves stroke risk prediction: usefulness of a new ultrasonographic score. Cerebrovasc Dis. 2011;31(3):300-4. PMID: 21212660.

103. Ranke C, Creutzig A, Becker H, et al. Standardization of carotid ultrasound: a hemodynamic method to normalize for interindividual and interequipment variability. Stroke. 1999;30(2):402-6. PMID: 9933279.

104. Reed AB, Gaccione P, Belkin M, et al. Preoperative risk factors for carotid endarterectomy: defining the patient at high risk. J Vasc Surg. 2003;37(6):1191-9. PMID: 12764264.

105. Reinhard M, Gerds TA, Grabiak D, et al. Cerebral dysautoregulation and the risk of ischemic events in occlusive carotid artery disease. J Neurol. 2008;255(8):1182-9.

106. Reiter M, Bucek RA, Effenberger I, et al. Plaque echolucency is not associated with the risk of stroke in carotid stenting. Stroke. 2006;37(9):2378-80. PMID: 16888264.

107. Rockman CB, Jacobowitz GR, Gagne PJ, et al. Focused screening for occult carotid artery disease: patients with known heart disease are at high risk. J Vasc Surg. 2004;39(1):44-51. PMID: 14718811.

108. Roh HG, Byun HS, Ryoo JW, et al. Prospective analysis of cerebral infarction after carotid endarterectomy and carotid artery stent placement by using diffusion-weighted imaging. AJNR Am J Neuroradiol. 2005;26(2):376-84. PMID: 15709140.

109. Roh YN, Woo SY, Kim N, et al. Prevalence of asymptomatic carotid stenosis in Korea based on health screening population. J Korean Med Sci. 2011;26(9):1173-7. PMID: 21935272.

110. Rosenthal DE. Carotid endarterectomy in the octogenarian: is it appropriate? J Vasc Surg. 1986;3(5).

111. Rothwell PM, Slattery J, Warlow CP. Clinical and angiographic predictors of stroke and death from carotid endarterectomy: systematic review. BMJ. 1997;315(7122):1571-7. PMID: 9437274.

112. Sahlein DH, Heyer EJ, Rampersad A, et al. Failure of intraoperative jugular bulb S-100B and neuron-specific enolase sampling to predict cognitive injury after carotid endarterectomy. Neurosurgery. 2003;53(6):1243-9. PMID: 14633290.

113. Samra SK, Dy EA, Welch K, et al. Evaluation of a cerebral oximeter as a monitor of cerebral ischemia during carotid endarterectomy. Anesthesiology. 2000;93(4):964-70. PMID: 11020747.

114. Schlager O, Exner M, Mlekusch W, et al. C-reactive protein predicts future cardiovascular events in patients with carotid stenosis. Stroke. 2007;38(4):1263-8. PMID: 17322087.

115. Schmidt P, Sliwka U, Simon SG, et al. High-grade stenosis of the internal carotid artery assessed by color and power Doppler imaging. J Clin Ultrasound. 1998;26(2):85-9. PMID: 9460636.

Appendix C. Excluded Studies

116. Sherif C, Dick P, Sabeti S, et al. Neurological outcome of conservative versus endovascular treatment of patients with asymptomatic high-grade carotid artery stenosis: a propensity score-adjusted analysis. J Endovasc Ther. 2005;12(2):145-55. PMID: 15823061.

117. Silvestrini M, Altamura C, Cerqua R, et al. Ultrasonographic markers of vascular risk in patients with asymptomatic carotid stenosis. J Cereb Blood Flow Metab. 2013;33(4):619-24. PMID: 23361391.

118. Skjelland M, Krohg-Sorensen K, Tennoe B, et al. Cerebral microemboli and brain injury during carotid artery endarterectomy and stenting. Stroke. 2009;40(1):230-4. PMID: 18927460.

119. Spence JD, Tamayo A, Lownie SP, et al. Absence of microemboli on transcranial Doppler identifies low-risk patients with asymptomatic carotid stenosis. Stroke. 2005;36(11):2373-8. PMID: 16224084.

120. Stoner MC, Abbott WM, Wong DR, et al. Defining the high-risk patient for carotid endarterectomy: an analysis of the prospective National Surgical Quality Improvement Program database. J Vasc Surg. 2006;43(2):285-95. PMID: 16476603.

121. Sutton-Tyrrell K, Alcorn HG, Wolfson SK Jr, et al. Predictors of carotid stenosis in older adults with and without isolated systolic hypertension. Stroke. 1993;24(3):355-61. PMID: 8446969.

122. Takaya N, Yuan C, Chu B, et al. Association between carotid plaque characteristics and subsequent ischemic cerebrovascular events: a prospective assessment with MRI—initial results. Stroke. 2006;37(3):818-23. PMID: 16469957.

123. Topakian R, King A, Kwon SU, et al. Ultrasonic plaque echolucency and emboli signals predict stroke in asymptomatic carotid stenosis. Neurology. 2011;77(8):751-8. PMID: 21849657.

124. van Lammeren GW, Moll FL, Blankestijn PJ, et al. Decreased kidney function: an unrecognized and often untreated risk factor for secondary cardiovascular events after carotid surgery. Stroke. 2011;42(2):307-12. PMID: 21183753.

125. Willeit J, Kiechl S, Santer P, et al. Lipoprotein(a) and asymptomatic carotid artery disease. Evidence of a prominent role in the evolution of advanced carotid plaques: the Bruneck Study. Stroke. 1995;26(9):1582-7. PMID: 7660402.

126. Wolf O, Heider P, Heinz M, et al. Microembolic signals detected by transcranial Doppler sonography during carotid endarterectomy and correlation with serial diffusion-weighted imaging. Stroke. 2004;35(11):e373-5. PMID: 15388901.

127. Yamada K, Yoshimura S, Kawasaki M, et al. Prediction of silent ischemic lesions after carotid artery stenting using virtual histology intravascular ultrasound. Cerebrovasc Dis. 2011;32(2):106-13. PMID: 21709408.

128. Yavas S, Mavioglu L, Kocabeyoglu S, et al. Is female gender really a risk factor for carotid endarterectomy? Ann Vasc Surg. 2010;24(6):775-85. PMID: 20471213.

129. Yuo TH, Goodney PP, Powell RJ, et al. "Medical high risk" designation is not associated with survival after carotid artery stenting. J Vasc Surg. 2008;47(2):356-62. PMID: 18155875.

130. Zahn RE. Carotid artery stenting in octogenarians: result from the ALKK Carotid Artery Stent (CAS) Registry. Eur Heart J. 2007;28.

Appendix D Table 1. Quality Ratings for Studies of Risk Stratification Tools (KQ 2)

First Author, Year	Overall attrition	Did the study have high attrition raising concern for bias?	Equal, valid, reliable ascertainment of exposure/ risk factors?	Equal, valid, reliable ascertainment of CAS?	Were assessors of CAS masked to risk factors?	Were multiple measures of performance used?	Was an appropriate method used to handle missing data?	Did the study use acceptable statistical methods?	If net reclassification was assessed, were appropriate clinical thresholds used to reclassify risk?	Was the sample size adequate to detect differences?	Quality Rating
Suri, 2008[1] Derivation cohorts: Jacobowitz, 2003[2] Qureshi, 2001[3]	2%	No	Yes	Yes	Yes	No	NA	Jacobowitz model: Yes Qureshi model: No*	NA	Yes	Jacobowitz model, 50% stenosis: Fair Jacobowitz model, 75% stenosis: Poor Qureshi model: Poor

* Everyone in the validation cohort was older than age 65 years, so the authors recreated the risk score without the age variable, and it had the highest weight/points in the original model.

Abbreviations: CAS = carotid artery stenosis; KQ = key question.

Appendix D Table 2. Quality Ratings for Systematic Reviews of Accuracy of Duplex Ultrasonography (KQ 3)

First Author, Year	Was the review based on a focused question of interest?	Was the literature search strategy clearly described?	Was there evidence of a substantial effort to search for all relevant research?	Were there explicit inclusion/ exclusion criteria for the selection of studies?	Did at least 2 people independently review studies?	Was the validity of included studies adequately assessed?	Was publication bias assessed?	Was heterogeneity assessed and addressed?	Was the approach used to synthesize the information adequate and appropriate?	Were the authors' conclusions supported by the evidence they presented?	Quality Rating
Jahromi, 2005[4]	Yes	Yes	Yes	Yes	Yes	Yes	No	Yes	Yes	Yes	Good
Nederkoorn, 2003[5]	Yes	No	No (searched only 1 database, and limited to 1994 to 2001)	Yes	Yes	No	No	Yes for positivity criteria; no for clinical heterogeneity	Yes	No	Fair
Blakely, 1995[6]	Yes	Yes	Yes	Yes	Yes	Yes	No	Yes	Yes	Yes	Good

Good: Recent, relevant review with comprehensive sources and search strategies, explicit and relevant selection criteria, standard appraisal of included studies, and valid conclusions.
Fair: Recent, relevant review that is not clearly biased but lacks comprehensive sources and search strategies.
Poor: Outdated, irrelevant, or biased review without systematic search for studies, explicit selection criteria, or standard appraisal of studies.

Appendix D Table 3. Quality Ratings for Primary Studies of Accuracy of Duplex Ultrasonography (KQ 3)

First Author, Year	Test(s) adequately described (or referenced)?	Was the spectrum of patients representative of the patients who will receive the test in PC?	Were selection criteria clearly described?	Is the reference standard likely to correctly classify the target condition?	Is the time period between the test and reference test short enough (to be reasonably sure that the condition did not change between the 2 tests)?	Did the whole or a random selection of the sample receive reference test?	Did patients receive the same reference regardless of test results?	Was the reference standard independent of the test?
Jogestrand, 2002[7]; Nowak, 2007[8]	Yes	No (all were symptomatic)	Yes	Yes	Yes	Yes	Yes	No
Sabeti, 2004[9]	Yes	NR/CND	Yes (consecutive patients who underwent angiography)	Yes	Yes	Yes	Yes	NR/CND
Hwang, 2003[10]	Yes	No (all were undergoing CEA)	No	Yes	Yes	Yes	Yes	NR/CND

First Author, Year	Was the execution of the test described in enough details to permit replication of the test?	Was the execution of the reference standard described in enough detail to permit replication?	Were the index test and reference standard results interpreted independently (blinded)?	Were the same clinical data available when the test results were interpreted as would be available when the test is used in practice?	Were uninterpretable results reported and handled in a reasonable manner?	Were withdrawals from the study explained (post-enrollment)?	Were methods for calculating accuracy clearly reported and valid?	Sample size? Small: <50 Medium: 50-100 Large: >100	Quality Rating
Jogestrand, 2002[7]; Nowak, 2007[8]	Yes	Yes	Yes	NR/CND	Yes	Yes	Yes	Large (161 patients recruited; 134 included in analyses; both arteries included)	Poor
Sabeti, 2004[9]	Yes	Yes	Yes	NR/CND	NR/CND	NA	Yes	Large (503 patients, 1006 arteries)	Fair
Hwang, 2003[10]	Yes	Yes	Yes	NR/CND	NR/CND	NA	Yes	Large (147 patients, 171 arteries)	Poor

Good: Evaluates relevant available screening test, uses a credible reference standard, interprets reference standard independently of screening test, reliability of test assessed, has few or handles indeterminate results in a reasonable manner, includes large number (>100) broad-spectrum patients with and without disease.
Fair: Evaluates relevant available screening test, uses reasonable although not best standard, interprets reference standard independent of screening test, moderate sample size (50-100 subjects), and a "medium" spectrum of patients.
Poor: Has fatal flaw such as uses inappropriate reference standard, screening test improperly administered, biased ascertainment of reference standard, very small sample size, or very narrowly selected spectrum of patients.

Abbreviations: CEA = carotid endarterectomy; CND = cannot determine; NR = not reported; PC = primary care.

Appendix D Table 4. Quality Ratings for Systematic Reviews and Meta-Analyses for Benefit of Treatment (KQ 5)

First Author, Year	Was the review based on a focused question of interest?	Was the literature search strategy clearly described?	Was there evidence of a substantial effort to search for all relevant research?	Were there explicit inclusion/exclusion criteria for the selection of studies?	Did at least 2 people independently review studies?	Was the validity of included studies adequately assessed?	Was publication bias assessed?	Was heterogeneity assessed and addressed?	Was the approach used to synthesize the information adequate and appropriate?	Were the authors' conclusions supported by the evidence they presented?	Quality Rating
Benavente, 1998[11]	Yes	Yes	Yes	Yes	Yes	No	No	Yes for statistical heterogeneity; no for clinical heterogeneity	No	No	Poor
Chambers, 2005[12]	Yes	Yes	Yes	Yes	Yes	Yes	No	Yes	Yes	Yes	Good
Wolff, 2007[13]; Wolff, 2007[14]	Yes	Yes	Yes	Yes	Yes for KQ 4; no for other KQs (they report that articles were selected for review and abstracted by 1 reviewer)	Yes	No	Yes	Yes	Yes	Fair
Raman, 2012[15]; Raman, 2013[16]	Yes	Yes	Yes	Yes	Yes	Yes	No	Yes	Yes	Yes	Good
Guay, 2012[17]	Yes	Yes, but just searched 1 database	Yes	Yes	No	Yes	No	No for clinical heterogeneity. They combined many studies with substantially different comparator groups	No; they combined many studies with substantially different comparator groups	Yes	Poor

Good: Recent, relevant review with comprehensive sources and search strategies; explicit and relevant selection criteria; standard appraisal of included studies; and valid conclusions.
Fair: Recent, relevant review that is not clearly biased but lacks comprehensive sources and search strategies.
Poor: Outdated, irrelevant, or biased review without systematic search for studies, explicit selection criteria, or standard appraisal of studies.

Abbreviation: KQ = key question.

Appendix D Table 5. Quality Ratings for Randomized, Controlled Trials for Benefit of Treatment (KQ 5)

Study, First Author, Year	Was randomization adequate?	Was allocation concealment adequate?	Were groups similar at baseline?	Was intervention fidelity adequate?	Was adherence to the intervention adequate?	What was the overall attrition*?	What was the differential attrition*?	Did the study have differential or overall high attrition raising concern for bias?
ACST, Halliday, 2004[18] Halliday, 2010[19] den Hartog, 2013[20] Halliday, 1994[21] Halliday, 1995[22]	Yes	Yes	Yes	Yes	Yes	5.8% immediate; 6.7% deferred; 1.9% (followup to death or at least year 3 was 98% complete; 3062/3120)	0.9%	No
ACAS, ACAS Study Group, 1995[23] Baker, 2000[24] Young, 1996[25]	Yes	Yes	Yes	Yes	Yes	1.2% (median followup, 2.7 y; 87% of patients completed 1 y of followup; 68% completed 2 y; 44% completed 3 y; 26% completed 4 y; and 9% completed 5 y)	0.1%	No
VACS, Towne, 1990[26] Hobson, 1993[27] Hobson 1986[28]	Yes	Yes	Yes	Yes	Yes	Surgery: 9.5% MM: 6.4% (Mean, 48 months of followup)	3.1%	No

* Attrition includes participants with no outcome data.

Study, First Author, Year	Did the study have crossovers or contamination raising concern for bias?	Were outcome measurements equal, valid and reliable?	Were outcome assessors masked?	Was the duration of followup adequate to assess the outcome?	Was an appropriate method used to handle missing data?	Did the study use acceptable statistical methods?	Quality Rating
ACST, Halliday, 2004[18] Halliday, 2010[19] den Hartog, 2013[20] Halliday, 1994[21] Halliday, 1995[22]	Yes (10% of immediate CEA group had not undergone CEA by 1 year; 7.5% had not by year 10; 26% [407/1560] of the MM/deferral group underwent CEA within 10 years; about two thirds of these were asymptomatic CEAs)	Yes	No for the initial outcome assessor (e.g., the surgeon doing the CEA was typically the person filling out event reports); yes for the Endpoints Committee who sought medical records when strokes were reported.	Yes	CND	Yes	Fair
ACAS, ACAS Study Group, 1995[23] Baker, 2000[24] Young, 1996[25]	No	Yes	No for the initial neurologist and surgeon (but patients also completed standardized TIA/stroke questionnaires at followups and were instructed to contact the coordinator for any problems); yes for the Endpoints Committee.	Yes	Yes	Yes	Good (for the 2.7-y data that were based on actual events; higher risk of bias for the 5-y estimates because just 9% had followup)
VACS, Towne, 1990[26] Hobson, 1993[27] Hobson 1986[28]	No (only 3.8% [8/211] of CEA group did not undergo surgery; no reporting of subjects in the medical group getting CEA)	Yes	No for the initial neurologist and vascular surgeon at each center; yes for the Endpoints Committee.	Yes	Yes	Yes	Good

Good: Meets all criteria: comparable groups are assembled initially and maintained throughout the study (followup ≥80%); reliable and valid measurement instruments are used and applied equally to the groups; interventions are spelled out clearly; all important outcomes are considered; and appropriate attention to confounders in analysis. In addition, for RCTs, intention to treat analysis is used.

Fair: Any or all of the following problems occur, without the fatal flaws noted in the "poor" category: generally comparable groups are assembled initially but some question remains whether some (although not major) differences occurred with followup; measurement instruments are acceptable (although not the best) and generally applied equally; some but not all important outcomes are considered; and some but not all potential confounders are accounted for. Intention to treat analysis is done for RCTs.

Poor: Any of the following fatal flaws exists: groups assembled initially are not close to being comparable or maintained throughout the study; unreliable or invalid measurement instruments are used or not applied at all equally among groups (including not masking outcome assessment); and key confounders are given little or no attention. For RCTs, intention to treat analysis is lacking.

Abbreviations: CEA = carotid endarterectomy; CND = could not determine; KQ = key question; MM = medical management; TIA = transient ischemic attack; RCT = randomized, controlled trial.

Appendix D Table 6. Quality Ratings for Randomized, Controlled Trials for Harms of Treatment (KQ 8)

Study, First Author, Year	Were harms prespecified and defined?	Were ascertainment techniques for harms adequately described?	Were ascertainment techniques for harms equal, valid, and reliable?	Was duration of followup adequate for harms assessment?	Harms quality rating	Comments
ACST, Halliday, 2004[18] Halliday, 2010[19] den Hartog, 2013[20] Halliday, 1994[21] Halliday, 1995[22]	Yes	Yes	Yes for death or major stroke, perhaps less so for minor stroke and myocardial infarction (without masking of providers making the initial assessments)	Yes	Fair	For perioperative morbidity, still no masking of initial outcome assessors; may introduce bias (some incentive to underreport harms for surgeons doing the procedure, as the design paper explains that those with unacceptably high morbidity and mortality may be asked not to enter any more patients)
ACAS, ACAS Study Group, 1995[23] Baker, 2000[24] Young, 1996[25]	Yes	Yes	Yes	Yes	Good	For perioperative morbidity, still no masking of initial outcome assessors; may introduce bias (some incentive to underreport harms for surgeons doing the procedure)
VACS, Towne, 1990[26] Hobson, 1993[27] Hobson 1986[28]	Yes	Yes	Yes	Yes	Good	For perioperative morbidity, still no masking of initial outcome assessors; may introduce bias (some incentive to underreport harms for surgeons doing the procedure)

Good: Meets all criteria: comparable groups are assembled initially and maintained throughout the study (followup ≥80%); reliable and valid measurement instruments are used and applied equally to the groups; interventions are spelled out clearly; all important outcomes are considered; and appropriate attention to confounders in analysis. In addition, for RCTs, intention to treat analysis is used.

Fair: Any or all of the following problems occur, without the fatal flaws noted in the "poor" category: generally comparable groups are assembled initially but some question remains whether some (although not major) differences occurred with followup; measurement instruments are acceptable (although not the best) and generally applied equally; some but not all important outcomes are considered; and some but not all potential confounders are accounted for. Intention to treat analysis is done for RCTs.

Poor: Any of the following fatal flaws exists: groups assembled initially are not close to being comparable or maintained throughout the study; unreliable or invalid measurement instruments are used or not applied at all equally among groups (including not masking outcome assessment); and key confounders are given little or no attention. For RCTs, intention to treat analysis is lacking.

Abbreviations: KQ = key question; RCT = randomized, controlled trial.

Appendix D Table 7. Quality Ratings for Other Studies for Harms of Treatment (KQ 8)

First Author, Year	Were eligibility criteria clearly described?	Were subjects representative of the overall source population?	Was the symptom status of subjects determined using valid and reliable methods?	What was the overall attrition?	Did the study have high attrition raising concern for bias?	Were outcome assessors masked?	Were outcomes prespecified/ defined and adequately described?	Were outcome measures valid and reliable?	Quality Rating	Comments
Kresowik, 2004[29]	Yes	Yes	Yes	0	No	No	Yes	Yes	Fair	May have missed nonfatal neurologic events occurring after discharge that did not result in another hospitalization; no comprehensive exam by neurologist for outcome assessment.
Kresowik, 2001[30]	Yes	Yes	Yes	0	No	No	Yes	Yes	Fair	May have missed nonfatal neurologic events occurring after discharge that did not result in another hospitalization; no comprehensive exam by neurologist for outcome assessment.
Bratzler, 1996[31]	Yes	Yes	Yes	0	No	No	Yes	Yes	Fair	May have missed nonfatal neurologic events occurring after discharge that did not result in another hospitalization; no comprehensive exam by neurologist for outcome assessment; definition of symptomatic CAS required documentation of past TIA or stroke in the distribution of the carotid being operated on; documented dizziness or syncope was not considered evidence of symptomatic CAS.
Cebul, 1998[32]	Yes	Yes	Yes	0	No	No	Yes	Yes	Fair	May have missed nonfatal neurologic events occurring after discharge that did not result in another hospitalization; no comprehensive exam by neurologist for outcome assessment; interrater reliability for determining indication for surgery (TIA, stroke, asympt, or nonspecific symptoms) of 77% (kappa 0.69)
Halm, 2007[33]; Halm, 2009[34]	Yes	Yes	Yes	10% of potentially eligible cases were excluded due to missing data	No	No	Yes	Yes	Fair	May have missed nonfatal neurologic events occurring after discharge that did not result in another hospitalization; no comprehensive exam by neurologist for outcome assessment. Data abstractors had to pass a series of quality assurances and interrater reliability tests. Data reported had kappa from 0.60 to 1.0.

Appendix D Table 7. Quality Ratings for Other Studies for Harms of Treatment (KQ 8)

First Author, Year	Were eligibility criteria clearly described?	Were subjects representative of the overall source population?	Was the symptom status of subjects determined using valid and reliable methods?	What was the overall attrition?	Did the study have high attrition raising concern for bias?	Were outcome assessors masked?	Were outcomes prespecified/ defined and adequately described?	Were outcome measures valid and reliable?	Quality Rating	Comments
Halm, 2003[35]; Rockman, 2005[36]; Halm, 2005[37]; Press, 2006[38]	Yes	Yes	Yes	0	No	No	Yes	Yes	Fair	May have missed readmissions to other hospitals (only included readmissions to the index hospital); data from 1 region of New York; no comprehensive exam by neurologist for outcome assessment.
Karp, 1998[39]	Yes	Yes	Yes	1.8%	No	No	Yes	Yes	Fair	May have missed nonfatal neurologic events occurring after discharge that did not result in another hospitalization; no comprehensive exam by neurologist for outcome assessment.
Kresowik, 2000[40]	Yes	Yes	Yes	0	No	No	Yes	Yes	Fair	May have missed nonfatal neurologic events occurring after discharge that did not result in another hospitalization; no comprehensive exam by neurologist for outcome assessment.
Giacovelli, 2010[41]	Yes	Yes	Unclear	0	No	No	Yes	Yes	Fair	Used present on admission symptom designations to determine symptom status at baseline; used ICD-9 codes only for outcome ascertainment; no supplementation with review of medical records; in-hospital outcomes only.
Vouyouka, 2012[42]	Yes	Yes	Unclear	0	No	No	Yes	Yes	Fair	Used present on admission symptom designations to determine symptom status at baseline; used ICD-9 codes only for outcome ascertainment; no supplementation with review of medical records; in-hospital outcomes only
McPhee, 2007[43]	Yes	Yes	No	0	No	No	Yes	Yes	Fair	Before 10/2004 no specific CAAS ICD-9 code existed, so required 2-step method to identify CAAS procedures, with potential for misclassification. Used ICD-9 codes only for outcome ascertainment; no supplementation with review of medical records; in-hospital outcomes only; potential for bias due to misclassification of symptom status and whether stroke was the indication or a perioperative harm.

Appendix D Table 7. Quality Ratings for Other Studies for Harms of Treatment (KQ 8)

First Author, Year	Were eligibility criteria clearly described?	Were subjects representative of the overall source population?	Was the symptom status of subjects determined using valid and reliable methods?	What was the overall attrition?	Did the study have high attrition raising concern for bias?	Were outcome assessors masked?	Were outcomes prespecified/ defined and adequately described?	Were outcome measures valid and reliable?	Quality Rating	Comments
McPhee, 2008[44]	Yes	Yes	No	0	No	No	Yes	Yes	Fair	Used ICD-9 codes only for outcome ascertainment; no supplementation with review of medical records; in-hospital outcomes only; potential for bias due to misclassification of symptom status and whether stroke was the indication or a perioperative harm.
Timaran, 2009[45]	Yes	Yes	No	0	No	No	Yes	Yes	Fair	Used ICD-9 codes only for outcome ascertainment; no supplementation with review of medical records; in-hospital outcomes only; potential for bias due to misclassification of symptom status and whether stroke was the indication or a perioperative harm.
Giles, 2010[46]	Yes	Yes	No	0	No	No	Yes	Yes	Fair	Used ICD-9 codes only for outcome ascertainment; no supplementation with review of medical records; in-hospital outcomes only; potential for bias due to misclassification of symptom status and whether stroke was the indication or a perioperative harm.
Young, 2011[47]	Yes	Yes	No	0	No	No	Yes	Yes	Fair	Used ICD-9 codes only for outcome ascertainment; no supplementation with review of medical records; in-hospital outcomes only; potential for bias due to misclassification of symptom status and whether stroke was the indication or a perioperative harm.
Horner, 2002[48]	Yes	Unclear	Unclear	NR	Unclear	No	Yes	Yes	Poor	High risk of selection bias and measurement bias. Supplemented outcome information with questionnaire, but no information is given on % of post-surgery questionnaires completed, and this was a key aspect of ascertaining events; no comprehensive exam by neurologist for outcome assessment. VA NSQIP protocol does not ask specifically about preoperative symptom status. Likely to underestimate harms.

Appendix D Table 7. Quality Ratings for Other Studies for Harms of Treatment (KQ 8)

First Author, Year	Were eligibility criteria clearly described?	Were subjects representative of the overall source population?	Was the symptom status of subjects determined using valid and reliable methods?	What was the overall attrition?	Did the study have high attrition raising concern for bias?	Were outcome assessors masked?	Were outcomes prespecified/ defined and adequately described?	Were outcome measures valid and reliable?	Quality Rating	Comments
Samsa, 2002[49]	Yes	Unclear	Unclear	NR	Unclear	No	Yes	Yes	Poor	High risk of selection bias and measurement bias. Supplemented outcome information with interview at day 30, but no information is given on % of questionnaires completed and this was a key aspect of ascertaining events;; no comprehensive exam by neurologist for outcome assessment; VA NSQIP protocol does not ask specifically about preop symptom status. Likely to underestimate harms.
Woo, 2010[50]	Yes	No	Unclear	NR	No	No, but they were independent of the treatment team	Yes	Yes	Poor	High risk of selection bias; required to have complete 30-day followup for cases to get into the database; and exclusion criteria for many people at higher risk of death and other complications that limited the included sample to about 5,000 asymptomatic patients out of about 10,000 CEAs identified; symptom status determined by claims data only; NSQIP does not collect information on results of preoperative imaging (CT/MRI); no comprehensive exam by neurologist for outcome assessment; does not capture outcome data from facilities that don't participate in NSQIP.
Garg, 2011[51]	Yes	No	Unclear	NR	No	No	Yes	Yes	Poor	High risk of selection bias; required to have complete 30-day followup for cases to get into the database; and exclusion criteria for many people at higher risk of death and other complications that limited the included sample; symptom status determined by claims data only; validity of ascertainment of symptom status is not clear; NSQIP does not collect information on results of preoperative imaging (CT/MRI); no comprehensive exam by neurologist for outcome assessment; does not capture outcome data from facilities that don't participate in NSQIP.

First Author, Year	Were eligibility criteria clearly described?	Were subjects representative of the overall source population?	Was the symptom status of subjects determined using valid and reliable methods?	What was the overall attrition?	Did the study have high attrition raising concern for bias?	Were outcome assessors masked?	Were outcomes prespecified/ defined and adequately described?	Were outcome measures valid and reliable?	Quality Rating	Comments
Wallaert, 2012[52]	Yes	Unclear	Unclear	NR/CND	No	No	Yes	Yes	Poor	High risk of selection bias and measurement bias; required to have complete 30-day followup; NSQIP does not collect information on results of preoperative imaging (CT/MRI); no comprehensive exam by neurologist for outcome assessment; does not capture outcome data from facilities that don't participate in NSQIP; potential misclassification of symptom status from only using CPT codes; NSQIP may underestimage the rate of MI as it may not include non-ST elevation MI.
Theiss, 2008[53]	Yes	NR/CND	Yes	NR/CND	NR/CND	No	Yes	CND	Poor	High risk of selection bias; reporting to registry is voluntary. Patients have to be registered prospectively, followed and documented until discharge or death; not clear how many cases were not completely documented and whether cases with missing data were excluded or how missing data was handled. Registry data does not extend beyond discharge.
Palombo, 2009[54]	Yes	CND	Yes	0	No	No	No	CND	Poor	High risk of selection bias and medium to high risk of measurement bias; unclear whether cases are representative of source population.
Micari, 2010[55]	Yes	CND	CND	0	No	No	Yes	Yes, independent neurologist evaluation	Poor	High risk of selection bias; high volume centers and experienced operators; unclear how the 198 subjects were selected for the registry; adequacy of outcome data NR; voluntary reporting to database; not clear how many cases were not completely documented and whether cases with missing data were excluded or how missing data was handled.
Menyhei, 2011[56]	Yes	CND	CND	0	No	No	No	CND	Poor	High risk of selection bias and measurement bias; data submission voluntary.

Appendix D Table 7. Quality Ratings for Other Studies for Harms of Treatment (KQ 8)

First Author, Year	Were eligibility criteria clearly described?	Were subjects representative of the overall source population?	Was the symptom status of subjects determined using valid and reliable methods?	What was the overall attrition?	Did the study have high attrition raising concern for bias?	Were outcome assessors masked?	Were outcomes prespecified/ defined and adequately described?	Were outcome measures valid and reliable?	Quality Rating	Comments
Lindstrom, 2012[57]	Yes	CND	CND	0	No	CND	Yes	Yes	Poor	High risk of selection bias; unclear how cases get into the national registry; completeness and representativeness of registry unclear.
Sidawy, 2009[58]	No	CND	NR	42% (CEA) 55% (CAAS)	Yes	NR	Yes	Yes	Poor	High risk of selection bias, mainly due to attrition; missing 30-day outcomes for about half of the subjects.
Jim, 2012[59]	No	CND	NR	NR	CND	NR	Yes	Yes	Poor	High risk of selection bias; only included subjects with complete 30-day outcomes, and other publications from this registry are clear that around half of subjects often have no 30-day outcomes.
CASANOVA study group, 1991[60]	Yes	CND	Yes	1%	No	Yes	Yes	Yes	Fair	Subjects from one arm of an RCT; unclear how representative subjects were of overall source population.
MACE study group, 1992[61]	Yes	CND	NR	0	No	Yes	Yes	Yes	Fair	Subjects from one arm of an RCT.
Fairman, 2007[62]	Yes	CND	Yes	0	No	Yes	Yes	Yes	Fair	
Gray, 2009[63]	Yes	CND	Yes	0	No	Yes	Yes	Yes	Fair	Stroke outcomes assessors were masked, but MI and death were reported by the sites.
Chaturvedi, 2010[64] Matsumura, 2010[65]	Yes	CND	Yes	0	No	Yes	Yes	Yes	Fair	
McKinlay, 2003[66], McKinlay, 2005[67], Zarins, 2009[68]	Yes	Unclear	Yes	18% enrolled and did not undergo treatment or did not complete 30-day followup visit; 26% did not complete independent neurological exam at 30 days	Yes	No	Yes	Yes	Poor	Unclear whether cases are representative of the source population, 46% of the cohort met at least one CMS-defined criteria of high risk for surgery (based on age or comorbidity). Participating principal investigators had to demonstrate a history of low complication rate with CEA or CAAS in order to participate.

Appendix D Table 7. Quality Ratings for Other Studies for Harms of Treatment (KQ 8)

First Author, Year	Were eligibility criteria clearly described?	Were subjects representative of the overall source population?	Was the symptom status of subjects determined using valid and reliable methods?	What was the overall attrition?	Did the study have high attrition raising concern for bias?	Were outcome assessors masked?	Were outcomes prespecified/ defined and adequately described?	Were outcome measures valid and reliable?	Quality Rating	Comments
Yadav, 2004[69]	Yes	Unclear	Unclear	0%	No	Yes	Yes	Yes	Fair	Unclear whether cases are representative of the source population. All participants had to have at least one "high risk" factor (e.g. age >80, contralateral stenosis). Highly selected surgeons and interventionalists; participating interventionalists had to demonstrate a low complication rate with CEA or CAAS in order to participate in the trial. Unclear whether symptom status was determined using valid and reliable methods.
Brott, 2010[70]; Silver, 2011[71]	Yes	Unclear	Yes	3%	No	Yes	Yes	Yes	Fair	Unclear whether cases are representative of the source population. A comprehensive training and credentialing process was required of participating interventionalists; only those with low complication rates were invited to participate in the study.
Hopkins, 2010[72]	No	Unclear	Unclear	3%	No	No	Yes	Yes	Fair	Unclear whether cases are representative of the source population.
Mercado, 2013[73]	Yes	Unclear	Yes	NR	Unclear	No	Yes	Unclear	Poor	High risk of selection bias and measurement bias; unclear how many procedures out of the total procedures done were included in the CARE registry and in this publication; unclear how much missing data they had; only 66% of patients got a postprocedure NIHSS assessment; unclear how outcomes were assessed for the other third of patients; not clear who was doing the assessments across sites and how they were determining the presence of outcomes when not using NIHSS; in-hospital events only.
Yuo, 2013[74]	Yes	Yes	Unclear	0	No	No	Yes	Yes	Fair	Used present on admission designations to determine symptom status at baseline; used ICD-9 codes only for outcome ascertainment; no supplementation with review of medical records; in-hospital outcomes only.

Appendix D Table 7. Quality Ratings for Other Studies for Harms of Treatment (KQ 8)

First Author, Year	Were eligibility criteria clearly described?	Were subjects representative of the overall source population?	Was the symptom status of subjects determined using valid and reliable methods?	What was the overall attrition?	Did the study have high attrition raising concern for bias?	Were outcome assessors masked?	Were outcomes prespecified/ defined and adequately described?	Were outcome measures valid and reliable?	Quality Rating	Comments
Schermerhorn, 2013[75]	No	CND	NR	NR	CND	NR	Yes	Yes (definitions are, but unclear how they were applied)	Poor	High risk of selection bias; only included subjects with complete 30-day outcomes and other publications from this registry are clear that around half of subjects often have no 30-day outcomes.
Fokkema, 2013[76]	Yes	No	Unclear	NR	Unclear	No	Yes	No	Poor	High risk of selection bias; required to have complete 30-day followup for cases to get into the database in other NSQIP publications (not explicitly stated in this article); NSQIP does not collect information on indication for surgery (symptom status), so limited in ability to stratify by symptom status accurately; for outcomes, cardiac events only included new Q-wave MI on EKG or cardiac arrest that necessitated CPR (only capturing the more severe events; not capturing non-Q-wave MI, for example); for stroke, not clear how people were assessed; no comprehensive exam by neurologist for outcome assessment; does not capture outcome data from facilities that don't participate in NSQIP.
Rajamani, 2012[77]	Yes	Unclear	Yes	NR	Unclear	No	No	Unclear	Poor	High risk of selection bias and measurement bias; unclear how many procedures out of the total procedures done were included in the CARE registry and in this publication; unclear how much missing data they had; unclear how outcomes were assessed (encouraged use of NIHSS, but unclear how often it was used); not clear who was doing the assessments across sites and how they were determining the presence of outcomes when not using NIHSS; in-hospital events only.

Good: Meets all criteria: comparable groups are assembled initially and maintained throughout the study (followup ≥80%); reliable and valid measurement instruments are used and applied equally to the groups; interventions are spelled out clearly; all important outcomes are considered; and appropriate attention to confounders in analysis. In addition, for RCTs, intention to treat analysis is used.
Fair: Any or all of the following problems occur, without the fatal flaws noted in the "poor" category: generally comparable groups are assembled initially but some question remains whether some (although not major) differences occurred with followup; measurement instruments are acceptable (although not the best) and generally applied equally; some but not all important outcomes are considered; and some but not all potential confounders are accounted for. Intention to treat analysis is done for RCTs.

Appendix D Table 7. Quality Ratings for Other Studies for Harms of Treatment (KQ 8)

Poor: Any of the following fatal flaws exists: groups assembled initially are not close to being comparable or maintained throughout the study; unreliable or invalid measurement instruments are used or not applied at all equally among groups (including not masking outcome assessment); and key confounders are given little or no attention. For RCTs, intention to treat analysis is lacking.

Abbreviations: CAAS = carotid angioplasty and stenting; CAS = carotid artery stenosis; CEA = carotid endarterectomy; CMS = Centers for Medicare & Medicaid Services; CND = could not determine; CPR = cardiopulmonary resuscitation; CPT = Current Procedural Terminology; CT = computed tomography; EKG = electrocardiography; ICD = International Classification of Diseases; KQ = key question; MI = myocardial infarction; MRI = magnetic resonance imaging; NR = not reported; NIHSS = National Institutes of Health Stroke Scale; NSQIP = National Surgical Quality Improvement Program; TIA = transient ischemic attack; RCT = randomized, controlled trial; VA = Department of Veterans Affairs.

Appendix D. References

1. Suri MF, Ezzeddine MA, Lakshminarayan K, et al. Validation of two different grading schemes to identify patients with asymptomatic carotid artery stenosis in general population. J Neuroimaging. 2008 Apr;18(2):142-7. PMID: 18380694.
2. Jacobowitz GR, Rockman CB, Gagne PJ, et al. A model for predicting occult carotid artery stenosis: screening is justified in a selected population. J Vasc Surg. 2003 Oct;38(4):705-9. PMID: 14560217.
3. Qureshi AI, Janardhan V, Bennett SE, et al. Who should be screened for asymptomatic carotid artery stenosis? Experience from the Western New York Stroke Screening Program. J Neuroimaging. 2001 Apr;11(2):105-11. PMID: 11296578.
4. Jahromi AS, Cina CS, Liu Y, et al. Sensitivity and specificity of color duplex ultrasound measurement in the estimation of internal carotid artery stenosis: a systematic review and meta-analysis. J Vasc Surg. 2005 Jun;41(6):962-72. PMID: 15944595.
5. Nederkoorn PJ, Graaf Y, Hunink M. Duplex ultrasound and magnetic resonance angiography compared with digital subtraction angiography in carotid artery stenosis: a systematic review (Structured abstract). Stroke. 2003;34(5):1324-31. PMID: DARE-12003000974.
6. Blakeley DD, Oddone EZ, Hasselblad V, et al. Noninvasive carotid artery testing. A meta-analytic review. Ann Intern Med. 1995;122(5):360-7.
7. Jogestrand T, Lindqvist M, Nowak J. Diagnostic performance of duplex ultrasonography in the detection of high grade internal carotid artery stenosis. Eur J Vasc Endovasc Surg. 2002 Jun;23(6):510-8. PMID: 12093067.
8. Nowak J, Jogestrand T. Duplex ultrasonography is an efficient diagnostic tool for the detection of moderate to severe internal carotid artery stenosis. Clin Physiol Funct Imaging. 2007 May;27(3):144-7. PMID: 17445064.
9. Sabeti S, Schillinger M, Mlekusch W, et al. Quantification of internal carotid artery stenosis with duplex US: comparative analysis of different flow velocity criteria. Radiology. 2004 Aug;232(2):431-9. PMID: 15286315.
10. Hwang CS, Liao KM, Lee JH, et al. Measurement of carotid stenosis: comparisons between duplex and different angiographic grading methods. J Neuroimaging. 2003 Apr;13(2):133-9. PMID: 12722495.
11. Benavente O, Moher D, Pham B. Carotid endarterectomy for asymptomatic carotid stenosis: a meta-analysis. BMJ. 1998 Nov 28;317(7171):1477-80. PMID: 9831572.
12. Chambers Brian R, Donnan G. Carotid endarterectomy for asymptomatic carotid stenosis. Cochrane Database Syst Rev. 2005(4)PMID: CD001923.
13. Wolff T, Guirguis-Blake J, Miller T, et al. Screening for Asymptomatic Carotid Artery Stenosis. Evidence Synthesis Number 50. AHRQ Publication No. 08-05102-EF-1. Agency for Healthcare Research and Quality, December 2007 Rockville, MD.
14. Wolff T, Guirguis-Blake J, Miller T, et al. Screening for carotid artery stenosis: an update of the evidence for the U.S. Preventive Services Task Force. Ann Intern Med. 2007 Dec 18;147(12):860-70. PMID: 18087057.
15. Raman G, Kitsios GD, Moorthy D, et al. Management of Asymptomatic Carotid Artery Stenosis. Technology Assessment Report. Project ID: CRDT0510. Prepared for the Agency for Healthcare Research and Quality by the Tufts Evidence-based Practice Center. Rockville, MD: August 27, 2012.
16. Raman G, Moorthy D, Hadar N, et al. Management Strategies for Asymptomatic Carotid Stenosis: A Systematic Review and Meta-analysis. Ann Intern Med. 2013 May 7;158(9):676-85. PMID: 23648949.
17. Guay J, Ochroch EA. Carotid endarterectomy plus medical therapy or medical therapy alone for carotid artery stenosis in symptomatic or asymptomatic patients: a meta-analysis (Structured abstract). Cardiothorac Vasc Anesth. 2012;26(5):835-44. PMID: DARE-12012043839.
18. Halliday A, Mansfield A, Marro J, et al. Prevention of disabling and fatal strokes by successful carotid endarterectomy in patients without recent neurological symptoms: randomised controlled trial. Lancet. 2004 May 8;363(9420):1491-502. PMID: 15135594.
19. Halliday A, Harrison M, Hayter E, et al. 10-year stroke prevention after successful carotid endarterectomy for asymptomatic stenosis (ACST-1): a multicentre randomised trial. Lancet. 2010 Sep 25;376(9746):1074-84. PMID: 20870099.
20. den Hartog AG, Halliday AW, Hayter E, et al. Risk of stroke from new carotid artery occlusion in the Asymptomatic Carotid Surgery Trial-1. Stroke. 2013 Jun;44(6):1652-9. PMID: 23632980.
21. Halliday AW, Thomas D, Mansfield A. The Asymptomatic Carotid Surgery Trial (ACST). Rationale and design. Steering Committee. Eur J Vasc Surg. 1994;8(6):703-10. PMID: CN-00109424.
22. Halliday AW, Thomas DJ, Mansfield AO. The asymptomatic carotid surgery trial (ACST). International angiology : a journal of the International Union of Angiology. 1995;14(1):18-20. PMID: CN-00117646.
23. Endarterectomy for asymptomatic carotid artery stenosis. Executive Committee for the Asymptomatic Carotid Atherosclerosis Study. JAMA. 1995 May 10;273(18):1421-8. PMID: 7723155.

24. Baker WH, Howard VJ, Howard G, et al. Effect of contralateral occlusion on long-term efficacy of endarterectomy in the asymptomatic carotid atherosclerosis study (ACAS). ACAS Investigators. Stroke. 2000 Oct;31(10):2330-4. PMID: 11022059.

25. Young B, Moore WS, Robertson JT, et al. An analysis of perioperative surgical mortality and morbidity in the asymptomatic carotid atherosclerosis study. Stroke. 1996;27(12):2216-24.

26. Towne JB, Weiss DG, Hobson RW. First phase report of cooperative Veterans Administration asymptomatic carotid stenosis study--operative morbidity and mortality. J Vasc Surg. 1990;11(2):252-8; discussion 8-9. PMID: CN-00065284.

27. Hobson RW, 2nd, Weiss DG, Fields WS, et al. Efficacy of carotid endarterectomy for asymptomatic carotid stenosis. The Veterans Affairs Cooperative Study Group. N Engl J Med. 1993 Jan 28;328(4):221-7. PMID: 8418401.

28. Role of carotid endarterectomy in asymptomatic carotid stenosis. A Veterans Administration Cooperative Study. Stroke; a journal of cerebral circulation. 1986;17(3):534-9. PMID: CN-00043144.

29. Kresowik Tea. Multistate improvement in process and outcomes of carotid endarterectomy. J Vasc Surg. 2004;39(2).

30. Kresowik TF, Bratzler D, Karp HR, et al. Multistate utilization, processes, and outcomes of carotid endarterectomy. J Vasc Surg. 2001 Feb;33(2):227-34; discussion 34-5. PMID: 11174772.

31. Bratzler DW, Oehlert WH, Murray CK, et al. Carotid endarterectomy in Oklahoma Medicare beneficiaries: patient characteristics and outcomes. J Okla State Med Assoc. 1996 Dec;89(12):423-9. PMID: 8997882.

32. Cebul RD, Snow RJ, Pine R, et al. Indications, outcomes, and provider volumes for carotid endarterectomy. JAMA. 1998 Apr 22-29;279(16):1282-7. PMID: 9565009.

33. Halm EA, Tuhrim S, Wang JJ, et al. Has evidence changed practice?: appropriateness of carotid endarterectomy after the clinical trials. Neurology. 2007 Jan 16;68(3):187-94. PMID: 17224571.

34. Halm EA, Tuhrim S, Wang JJ, et al. Risk factors for perioperative death and stroke after carotid endarterectomy: results of the new york carotid artery surgery study. Stroke. 2009 Jan;40(1):221-9. PMID: 18948605.

35. Halm EA, Chassin MR, Tuhrim S, et al. Revisiting the appropriateness of carotid endarterectomy. Stroke. 2003 Jun;34(6):1464-71. PMID: 12738896.

36. Rockman CB, Halm EA, Wang JJ, et al. Primary closure of the carotid artery is associated with poorer outcomes during carotid endarterectomy. J Vasc Surg. 2005 Nov;42(5):870-7. PMID: 16275440.

37. Halm EA, Hannan EL, Rojas M, et al. Clinical and operative predictors of outcomes of carotid endarterectomy. J Vasc Surg. 2005 Sep;42(3):420-8. PMID: 16171582.

38. Press MJ, Chassin MR, Wang J, et al. Predicting medical and surgical complications of carotid endarterectomy: comparing the risk indexes. Arch Intern Med. 2006 Apr 24;166(8):914-20. PMID: 16636219.

39. Karp HR, Flanders WD, Shipp CC, et al. Carotid endarterectomy among Medicare beneficiaries: a statewide evaluation of appropriateness and outcome. Stroke. 1998 Jan;29(1):46-52. PMID: 9445327.

40. Kresowik TF, Hemann RA, Grund SL, et al. Improving the outcomes of carotid endarterectomy: results of a statewide quality improvement project. J Vasc Surg. 2000 May;31(5):918-26. PMID: 10805882.

41. Giacovelli JK, Egorova N, Dayal R, et al. Outcomes of carotid stenting compared with endarterectomy are equivalent in asymptomatic patients and inferior in symptomatic patients. J Vasc Surg. 2010 Oct;52(4):906-13, 13 e1-4. PMID: 20620010.

42. Vouyouka AG, Egorova NN, Sosunov EA, et al. Analysis of Florida and New York state hospital discharges suggests that carotid stenting in symptomatic women is associated with significant increase in mortality and perioperative morbidity compared with carotid endarterectomy. J Vasc Surg. 2012 Aug;56(2):334-42. PMID: 22583852.

43. McPhee JT, Hill JS, Ciocca RG, et al. Carotid endarterectomy was performed with lower stroke and death rates than carotid artery stenting in the United States in 2003 and 2004. J Vasc Surg. 2007 Dec;46(6):1112-8. PMID: 18154987.

44. McPhee JT, Schanzer A, Messina LM, et al. Carotid artery stenting has increased rates of postprocedure stroke, death, and resource utilization than does carotid endarterectomy in the United States, 2005. J Vasc Surg. 2008 Dec;48(6):1442-50, 50 e1. PMID: 18829236.

45. Timaran CH, Veith FJ, Rosero EB, et al. Intracranial hemorrhage after carotid endarterectomy and carotid stenting in the United States in 2005. J Vasc Surg. 2009 Mar;49(3):623-8; discussion 8-9. PMID: 19268766.

46. Giles KA, Hamdan AD, Pomposelli FB, et al. Stroke and death after carotid endarterectomy and carotid artery stenting with and without high risk criteria. J Vasc Surg. 2010 Dec;52(6):1497-504. PMID: 20864299.

47. Young KC, Jahromi BS. Does current practice in the United States of carotid artery stent placement benefit asymptomatic octogenarians? AJNR Am J Neuroradiol. 2011 Jan;32(1):170-3. PMID: 20864521.

48. Horner RD, Oddone EZ, Stechuchak KM, et al. Racial variations in postoperative outcomes of carotid endarterectomy: evidence from the Veterans Affairs National Surgical Quality Improvement Program. Med Care. 2002 Jan;40(1 Suppl):I35-43. PMID: 11789630.

49. Samsa G, Oddone EZ, Horner R, et al. To what extent should quality of care decisions be based on health outcomes data? Application to carotid endarterectomy. Stroke. 2002 Dec;33(12):2944-9. PMID: 12468795.

50. Woo K, Garg J, Hye RJ, et al. Contemporary results of carotid endarterectomy for asymptomatic carotid stenosis. Stroke. 2010 May;41(5):975-9. PMID: 20339122.

51. Garg J, Frankel DA, Dilley RB. Carotid endarterectomy in academic versus community hospitals: the national surgical quality improvement program data. Ann Vasc Surg. 2011 May;25(4):433-41. PMID: 21435832.

52. Wallaert JB, De Martino RR, Finlayson SR, et al. Carotid endarterectomy in asymptomatic patients with limited life expectancy. Stroke. 2012 Jul;43(7):1781-7. PMID: 22550053.

53. Theiss W, Hermanek P, Mathias K, et al. Predictors of death and stroke after carotid angioplasty and stenting: a subgroup analysis of the Pro-CAS data. Stroke. 2008 Aug;39(8):2325-30. PMID: 18583556.

54. Palombo D, Lucertini G, Mambrini S, et al. Carotid endarterectomy: results of the Italian Vascular Registry. J Cardiovasc Surg (Torino). 2009 Apr;50(2):183-7. PMID: 19282808.

55. Micari A, Stabile E, Cremonesi A, et al. Carotid artery stenting in octogenarians using a proximal endovascular occlusion cerebral protection device: a multicenter registry. Catheter Cardiovasc Interv. 2010 Jul 1;76(1):9-15. PMID: 20578188.

56. Menyhei G, Bjorck M, Beiles B, et al. Outcome following carotid endarterectomy: lessons learned from a large international vascular registry. Eur J Vasc Endovasc Surg. 2011 Jun;41(6):735-40. PMID: 21450496.

57. Lindstrom D, Jonsson M, Formgren J, et al. Outcome after 7 years of carotid artery stenting and endarterectomy in Sweden - single centre and national results. Eur J Vasc Endovasc Surg. 2012 May;43(5):499-503. PMID: 22342694.

58. Sidawy AN, Zwolak RM, White RA, et al. Risk-adjusted 30-day outcomes of carotid stenting and endarterectomy: results from the SVS Vascular Registry. J Vasc Surg. 2009 Jan;49(1):71-9. PMID: 19028045.

59. Jim J, Rubin BG, Ricotta JJ, 2nd, et al. Society for Vascular Surgery (SVS) Vascular Registry evaluation of comparative effectiveness of carotid revascularization procedures stratified by Medicare age. J Vasc Surg. 2012 May;55(5):1313-20; discussion 21. PMID: 22459755.

60. Carotid surgery versus medical therapy in asymptomatic carotid stenosis. The CASANOVA Study Group. Stroke. 1991 Oct;22(10):1229-35. PMID: 1926232.

61. Wiebers DO, Whisnant JP, Meissner I, et al. Results of a randomized controlled trial of carotid endarterectomy for asymptomatic carotid stenosis. Mayo Clin Proc. 1992;67(6):513-8.

62. Fairman R, Gray WA, Scicli AP, et al. The CAPTURE registry: analysis of strokes resulting from carotid artery stenting in the post approval setting: timing, location, severity, and type. Ann Surg. 2007 Oct;246(4):551-6; discussion 6-8. PMID: 17893491.

63. Gray WA, Chaturvedi S, Verta P. Thirty-day outcomes for carotid artery stenting in 6320 patients from 2 prospective, multicenter, high-surgical-risk registries. Circ Cardiovasc Interv. 2009 Jun;2(3):159-66. PMID: 20031712.

64. Chaturvedi S, Matsumura JS, Gray W, et al. Carotid artery stenting in octogenarians: periprocedural stroke risk predictor analysis from the multicenter Carotid ACCULINK/ACCUNET Post Approval Trial to Uncover Rare Events (CAPTURE 2) clinical trial. Stroke. 2010 Apr;41(4):757-64. PMID: 20185789.

65. Matsumura JS, Gray W, Chaturvedi S, et al. CAPTURE 2 risk-adjusted stroke outcome benchmarks for carotid artery stenting with distal embolic protection. J Vasc Surg. 2010 Sep;52(3):576-83, 83 e1-83 e2. PMID: 20576398.

66. CaRESS Steering Committee. Carotid revascularization using endarterectomy or stenting systems (CARESS): Phase I clinical trial. J Endovasc Ther. 2003 Dec;10(6):1021-30. PMID: 14723574.

67. McKinlay SM. Carotid Revascularization Using Endarterectomy or Stenting Systems (CaRESS) phase I clinical trial: 1-Year results. J Vasc Surg. 2005;42(2):213-9.

68. Zarins CK, White RA, Diethrich EB, et al. Carotid revascularization using endarterectomy or stenting systems (CaRESS): 4-year outcomes. J Endovasc Ther. 2009 Aug;16(4):397-409. PMID: 19702339.

69. Yadav JS, Wholey MH, Kuntz RE, et al. Protected carotid-artery stenting versus endarterectomy in high-risk patients. N Engl J Med. 2004 Oct 7;351(15):1493-501. PMID: 15470212.

70. Brott TG, Hobson RW, 2nd, Howard G, et al. Stenting versus endarterectomy for treatment of carotid-artery stenosis. N Engl J Med. 2010 Jul 1;363(1):11-23. PMID: 20505173.

Appendix D. References

71. Silver FL, Mackey A, Clark WM, et al. Safety of stenting and endarterectomy by symptomatic status in the Carotid Revascularization Endarterectomy Versus Stenting Trial (CREST). Stroke. 2011 Mar;42(3):675-80. PMID: 21307169.

72. Hopkins LN, Roubin GS, Chakhtoura EY, et al. The Carotid Revascularization Endarterectomy versus Stenting Trial: credentialing of interventionalists and final results of lead-in phase. Journal of stroke and cerebrovascular diseases : the official journal of National Stroke Association. 2010;19(2):153-62. PMID: CN-00751863.

73. Mercado N, Cohen DJ, Spertus JA, et al. Carotid artery stenting of a contralateral occlusion and in-hospital outcomes: results from the CARE (Carotid Artery Revascularization and Endarterectomy) registry. JACC Cardiovasc Interv. 2013 Jan;6(1):59-64. PMID: 23347862.

74. Yuo TH, Degenholtz HS, Chaer RA, et al. Effect of hospital-level variation in the use of carotid artery stenting versus carotid endarterectomy on perioperative stroke and death in asymptomatic patients. J Vasc Surg. 2013 Mar;57(3):627-34. PMID: 23312937.

75. Schermerhorn ML, Fokkema M, Goodney P, et al. The impact of Centers for Medicare and Medicaid Services high-risk criteria on outcome after carotid endarterectomy and carotid artery stenting in the SVS Vascular Registry. J Vasc Surg. 2013 May;57(5):1318-24. PMID: 23406712.

76. Fokkema M, Bensley RP, Lo RC, et al. In-hospital versus postdischarge adverse events following carotid endarterectomy. J Vasc Surg. 2013 Jun;57(6):1568-75, 75 e1-3. PMID: 23388394.

77. Rajamani K, Kennedy KF, Ruggiero NJ, et al. Outcomes of carotid endarterctomy in the elderly: A report from the care registry(registered trademark). Stroke. 2012;43(2).

Appendix E Table 1. Accuracy of Screening With Duplex Ultrasonography to Detect CAS (KQ 3)

First author, Year	Study Design	N	Degree of Stenosis	Method of Classification	Proportion of Arteries Asymptomatic	Mean Age	% Men	Sensitivity (95% CI)	Specificity (95% CI)	Quality
Nowak, 2007[1]; Jogestrand, 2002[2]	Prospective	134	≥70%; PSV=230 cm/s ≥80%; PSV=260 cm/s	ECST	NR	69 y	66	92% (89% to 95%) 88% (85% to 91%)	91% (87% to 95%) 86% (83% to 89%)	Poor
Jahromi, 2005[3a]	SR/MA	1,716 2,140	≥50%; PSV ≥130 cm/s ≥70%; PSV ≥200 cm/s	NASCET	NR	66 y	70	98% (97% to 100%) 90% (84% to 94%)	88% (76% to 100%) 94% (88% to 97%)	Good
Nederkoorn, 2003[4a]	SR/MA	NR	70% to 99%	NASCET	NR	NR	NR	86% (84% to 89%)	87% (84% to 90%)	Fair
Blakely, 1995[5]	SR/MA	3,989 2,646	>50% >70%	NASCET	NR	62 y	65	91% (85% to 93%)[b] 88% (83% to 91%)[b]	92% (88% to 93%)[b] 91% (87% to 94%)[b]	Good
Hwang, 2003[6]	Cross-sectional	171	≥70%	NASCET ECST CC	NR	68 y	65	96% 91% 92%	29% 70% 89%	Poor
Wolff, 2007[7]; Wolff, 2007[8c]	SR	NR	60% to 99%	NR	NR	NR	NR	94%	92%	Fair
Sabeti, 2004[9]	Cross-sectional	1,006	70% to 99%; PSV>250 cm/s	NASCET	NR	70 y	69	97% (95% to 99%)	66% (63% to 71%)	Fair

[a] Used as evidence in the 2007 comparative effectiveness review.
[b] Values estimated from figure.
[c] 2007 comparative effectiveness review and associated *Annals in Internal Medicine* article.

Abbreviations: CC = common carotid; CI = confidence interval; ECST = European Carotid Surgery Trial; KQ = key question; MA = meta-analysis; N = sample size; NASCET = North American Symptomatic Carotid Endarterectomy Trial; NR = not reported; PSV = peak systolic velocity; RCT = randomized, controlled trial; SR = systematic review.

Study, Year	Study Design & Period	Procedure N total (N Asymp)	Setting, Source Population[b]	Sample Selection Criteria	Sample Subjects' Characteristics[a]	Threats to Internal and External Validity	Quality
Horner, 2002[10]	Cohort study 10/1994-9/1997	CEA 6,551 (2,852; 140 black, 93 Hispanic, 2,619 white)	VA NSQIP[b] database CEA cases searched by CPT code	CPT codes to identify men who underwent CEA. Women were excluded from this analysis. Asymptomatic status defined by excluding codes related to TIA or stroke.	Age ≥75 y: 18% (black), 20% (Hispanic), 20% (white) White: 91% Female: 0% DM: 27% (black), 36% (Hispanic), 21% (white) CAD: NR COPD (severe): 7% (black), 11% (Hispanic), 21% (white) HF: 2% (black), 1% (Hispanic), 2% (white) HTN: NR Smoker: NR Stenosis: NR Prior contralateral CEA: NR Contralateral occlusion: NR Contralateral Stroke/TIA: NR	High risk of selection bias and measurement bias. Supplemented outcome information with questionnaire, but no information is given on % of post-surgery questionnaires completed, and this was a key aspect of ascertaining events; no comprehensive exam by neurologist for outcome assessment. VA NSQIP protocol does not ask specifically about preoperative symptom status. Likely to underestimate harms.	Poor
Samsa, 2002[11]	Cohort study 1994-1997	CEA 7,842 (2,970)	VA NSQIP database Comparing event rates at VA medical centers with high complication rates by year (1994-1995 vs. 1996-1997)	CPT codes to identify patients who underwent CEA. Asymptomatic status defined by excluding codes related to TIA or stroke.	Mean Age: 68 y[c] White: 91% Female: 2% DM: 17% CAD: NR COPD: 17% HF: 2% HTN: NR Smoker: NR Stenosis: NR Prior contralateral CEA: NR Contralateral occlusion: NR Contralateral TIA/stroke: NR (only presence of any stroke/TIA)	High risk of selection bias and measurement bias. Supplemented outcome information with interview at day 30, but no information is given on % of questionnaires completed and this was a key aspect of ascertaining events; no comprehensive exam by neurologist for outcome assessment; VA NSQIP protocol does not ask specifically about preop symptom status. Likely to underestimate harms.	Poor
Woo, 2010[12]	Cohort study 2005-2007	CEA 5,009 (all asymptomatic)	NSQIP database	Trained clinical nurse reviewers input data from participating institutions. Asymptomatic status defined by excluding codes related to stroke and TIA.	Mean age: 71 y White: NR Female: 43% DM: 27% CAD: 1% with MI in prior 6 months, 25% with prior cardiac surgery COPD: 9% HF: <1% with HF within 30 days HTN: 86% Smoker: 25% (smoker within 1 year) Stenosis: NR prior contralateral CEA: NR contralateral occlusion: NR contralateral TIA/stroke: NR	High risk of selection bias; required to have complete 30-day followup for cases to get into the database; and exclusion criteria for many people at higher risk of death and other complications that limited the included sample to about 5,000 asymptomatic patients out of about 10,000 CEAs identified; symptom status determined by claims data only; NSQIP does not collect information on results of preoperative imaging (CT/MRI); no comprehensive exam by neurologist for outcome assessment; does not capture outcome data from facilities that don't participate in NSQIP.	Poor

Appendix E Table 2. Characteristics of Additional Studies Rated as Poor Quality and Reporting Rates of Periprocedural Complications of CEA or CAAS for Adults With Asymptomatic CAS

Study, Year	Study Design & Period	Procedure N total (N Asymp)	Setting, Source Population	Sample Selection Criteria	Sample Subjects' Characteristics[a]	Threats to Internal and External Validity	Quality
Garg,[13] 2011	Cohort study 2005-2009	CEA 17,388 (9,285)	NSQIP database	Trained clinical nurse reviewers input data from participating institutions. Asymptomatic status defined by excluding codes related to stroke and TIA.	Mean age: 71 y White: NR Female: 42% DM: 27% CAD: 1% (MI within 6 months); 19% (previous PTCA), 24% (previous cardiac surgery) COPD: 9% HF: <1% (within 1 month) HTN: 85% Smoker: 26% Stenosis: NR Prior contralateral CEA: NR Contralateral occlusion: NR Contralateral TIA/stroke: NR	High risk of selection bias; required to have complete 30-day followup for cases to get into the database; and exclusion criteria for many people at higher risk of death and other complications that limited the included sample; symptom status determined by claims data only; validity of ascertainment of symptom status is not clear; NSQIP does not collect information on results of preoperative imaging (CT/MRI); no comprehensive exam by neurologist for outcome assessment; does not capture outcome data from facilities that don't participate in NSQIP.	Poor
Wallaert,[14] 2012	Cohort study 2007-2009	CEA 22,696 (12,631) Analysis restricted to asymptomatic	NSQIP database	Asymptomatic status defined by excluding codes related to stroke and TIA. Study is evaluating 30-day event rates in people with life-limiting conditions.	Mean age: 72 y[d] White: 43% Female: 43% DM: 29% CAD: 42% COPD: NR HF: NR HTN: 86% Smoker: 29% Stenosis: NR Prior contralateral CEA: NR Contralateral occlusion: NR Contralateral TIA/stroke: NR	Unclear whether NSQIP subjects were representative of source population and how complete the sampling is; required to have complete 30-day followup; NSQIP does not collect information on results of preoperative imaging (CT/MRI); no comprehensive exam by neurologist for outcome assessment; does not capture outcome data from facilities that don't participate in NSQIP; potential misclassification of symptom status from only using CPT codes; NSQIP may underestimate the rate of MI as it may not include non-ST elevation MI.	Poor
Fokkema,[15] 2013	Cohort study 2005-2010	CEA 35,916 (~20,113)	NSQIP database	Asymptomatic patients defined as those with no history of stroke, TIA, or hemiplegia	Mean age: 72 y White: 92% Female: 41% DM: 28% CAD: NR COPD: 11% HF: 1% HTN: 85% Smoker: 28% Stenosis: NR Prior contralateral CEA: NR Contralateral occlusion: NR Contralateral TIA/stroke: NR	High risk of selection bias; required to have complete 30-day followup for cases to get into the database in other NSQIP publications (not explicitly stated in this article); NSQIP does not collect information on indication for surgery (symptom status), so limited in ability to stratify by symptom status accurately; for outcomes, cardiac events only included new Q-wave MI on EKG or cardiac arrest that necessitated CPR (only capturing the more severe events; not capturing non-Q-wave MI, for example); for stroke, not clear how people were assessed; no comprehensive exam by neurologist	Poor

Appendix E Table 2. Characteristics of Additional Studies Rated as Poor Quality and Reporting Rates of Periprocedural Complications of CEA or CAAS for Adults With Asymptomatic CAS

Study, Year	Study Design & Period	Procedure N total (N Asymp)	Setting, Source Population	Sample Selection Criteria	Sample Subjects' Characteristics[a]	Threats to Internal and External Validity	Quality
						for outcome assessment; does not capture outcome data from facilities that don't participate in NSQIP.	
Theiss, 2008[16]	Cohort study 7/1999-6/2005	CAAS 5,333 (2,412)	Pro-CAS database (Germany, Austria, Switzerland)	European (Pro-CAS) database: patients registered voluntarily by interventionist 24 hours before planned CAAS.	Median age: 70 y White: NR Female: 29% DM: NR CAD: NR COPD: NR HF: NR HTN: NR Smoker: NR Stenosis: NR Prior contralateral CEA: NR Contralateral occlusion: 23.7% had >90% occlusion Contralateral TIA/stroke: NR	High risk of selection bias; reporting to registry is voluntary. Patients have to be registered prospectively, followed and documented until discharge or death; not clear how many cases were not completely documented and whether cases with missing data were excluded or how missing data was handled. Registry data does not extend beyond discharge.	Poor
Palombo, 2009[17]	Cohort study 1/2007-12/2007	5,962 CEAs (4,068) 5,809 patients (NR)	Italian Registry for Vascular Activity	Italian registry of open surgical and endovascular activities of the centers fully dedicated to vascular surgery in Italy. Asymptomatic defined as no report of amaurosis fugax, TIA, or stroke in 6 months prior to surgery	Mean age: 73 y White: NR Female: 27.6% DM: 31% CAD: 53.4% COPD: NR HF: NR HTN: 89.7% Smoker: 70.7% Stenosis: ≥70% (98% of patients) Prior contralateral CEA: NR Contralateral occlusion: NR Contralateral TIA/stroke: NR	High risk of selection bias and medium to high risk of measurement bias; unclear whether cases are representative of source population.	Poor
Micari, 2010[18]	Cohort study 7/2005-5/2009	CAAS 198 (120)	Italian database; 3 institutions	Population includes consecutive octogenarians undergoing CAAS in 3 Italian centers	Median age: 83 y White: NR Female: 32% DM: 22% CAD: NR COPD: NR HF: NR HTN: 89% Smoker: 42% Stenosis: 100% of asymptomatic had ≥80% Prior contralateral CEA: NR Contralateral occlusion: 6% Contralateral TIA/stroke: NR	High risk of selection bias; high volume centers and experienced operators; unclear how the 198 subjects were selected for the registry; adequacy of outcome data NR; voluntary reporting to database; not clear how many cases were not completely documented and whether cases with missing data were excluded or how missing data was handled.	Poor

Appendix E Table 2. Characteristics of Additional Studies Rated as Poor Quality and Reporting Rates of Periprocedural Complications of CEA or CAAS for Adults With Asymptomatic CAS

Study, Year	Study Design & Period	Procedure N total (N Asymp)	Setting, Source Population	Sample Selection Criteria	Sample Subjects' Characteristics[a]	Threats to Internal and External Validity	Quality
Menyhei, 2011[19]	Cohort study 1/2003-12/2007	CEA 48,035 (NR; symptom status only reported on subset of included patients; 4,686 out of 18,034 were asymptomatic)	International registry (Vascunet); primarily European, but also includes Australia and New Zealand. 10 countries; not all had int/ext validation	Vascunet is a voluntary vascular registry collaboration	Median age: 67 y White: NR Female: 32% DM: NR CAD: NR COPD: NR HF: NR HTN: NR Smoker: NR Stenosis: NR Prior contralateral CEA: NR Contralateral occlusion: 9% Contralateral TIA/stroke: NR	High risk of selection bias and measurement bias; data submission voluntary.	Poor
Lindstrom, 2012[20]	Cohort study	CEA and CAAS CEA 6,474 (1,315) CAAS 258 (101)	Swedish Vascular Registry (Swedvasc)	Patients from entire country treated with CEA or CAAS; asymptomatic defined as no symptoms within last 180 days	CAAS:[e] Median age: 70 y White: NR Female: 30% DM: 29% CAD: 50% COPD: 14% HF: NR HTN: 81% Smoker: 70% Stenosis: NR Prior contralateral CEA: NR Contralateral occlusion: NR Contralateral TIA/stroke: ~45% asx	High risk of selection bias; unclear how cases get into the national registry; completeness and representativeness of registry unclear	Poor
Sidawy, 2009[21]	Cohort study 7/2005-12/2007	Full sample: CAAS 2,763 (1,404) CEA 3,259 (1,877) Patients with 30-day outcomes CAAS: 1,450 (805) CEA 1,368 (862)	Society for Vascular Surgery Vascular Registry (SVS-VR)	Online voluntary vascular surgery registry with audit program No specific inclusion or exclusion criteria	CAAS/CEA Mean age: 71/71 White: 94%/95% Female: 41%/40% DM: 33%/26% CAD: 61%/46% COPD: 18%/12% HF: 15%/7% HTN: 82%/79% Smoker: 59%/56% Stenosis: NR Prior contralateral CEA: NR Contralateral occlusion: NR Contralateral TIA/stroke: NR	High risk of selection bias, mainly due to attrition; missing 30-day outcomes for about half of the subjects	Poor

Appendix E Table 2. Characteristics of Additional Studies Rated as Poor Quality and Reporting Rates of Periprocedural Complications of CEA or CAAS for Adults With Asymptomatic CAS

Study, Year	Study Design & Period	Procedure N total (N Asymp)	Setting, Source Population	Sample Selection Criteria	Sample Subjects' Characteristics[a]	Threats to Internal and External Validity	Quality
Schermer-horn, 2013[22]	Cohort study 11/2001-9/2011	CAAS and CEA CAAS 3,737 (2,037) CEA 6,370 (3,964)	Society for Vascular Surgery Vascular Registry (SVS-VR)	Online voluntary vascular surgery registry with audit program No specific inclusion or exclusion criteria	CAAS/CEA Mean age: 71/71 y White: 92%/93% Female: 40%/31% DM: 34%/31% CAD: 58%/48% COPD: 20%/18% HF: 14%/8% HTN: 83%/84% Smoker: 61%/61% Stenosis: NR Prior contralateral CEA: NR Contralateral occlusion: 13%/4% Contralateral TIA/stroke: NR	High risk of selection bias; only included subjects with complete 30-day outcomes and other publications from this registry are clear in that around half of subjects often have no 30-day outcomes.	Poor
Jim, 2012[23]	Cohort study 7/2005-12/2010	CEA 5,516 (2,098) CAAS 3,397 (1,850)	SVS-VR	Online voluntary vascular surgery registry with audit program; results stratified by age (<65 and ≥65)	CEA<65/CAS<65 Mean age: 58/58 y White: 90%/89% Female: 40%/41% DM: 32%/36% CAD: 42%/52% COPD: 17%/20% HF: 6%/12% HTN: 81%/79% Smoker: 73%/69% Stenosis: NR Prior contralateral CEA: NR Contralateral occlusion: NR Contralateral TIA/stroke: NR

CEA≥65/CAS≥65 Mean age: 75/75 y White: 94%/93% Female: 42%/40% DM: 31%/32% CAD: 50%/61% COPD: 18%/20% HF: 9%/15% HTN: 85%/84% Smoker: 56%/57% Stenosis: NR Prior contralateral CEA: NR Contralateral occlusion: NR Contralateral TIA/stroke: NR | High risk of selection bias; only included subjects with complete 30-day outcomes and other publications fom this registry are clear in that around half of subjects often have no 30-day outcomes. | Poor |

Appendix E Table 2. Characteristics of Additional Studies Rated as Poor Quality and Reporting Rates of Periprocedural Complications of CEA or CAAS for Adults With Asymptomatic CAS

Study, Year	Study Design & Period	Procedure N total (N Asymp)	Setting, Source Population	Sample Selection Criteria	Sample Subjects' Characteristics[a]	Threats to Internal and External Validity	Quality
Mercado, 2013[24]	Cohort study 4/2005-1/2012	CAAS Full sample 13,993 (NR) Propensity-matched (analyzed) cohort 5,500 (3,048) CCO/No CCO 1,375 (763)/ 4,125 (2,285)	Carotid Artery Revascular-ization and Endarterect-omy (CARE) registry	Nationwide voluntary, hospital-based prospective database; patients considered asymptomatic if no history of any of the following: carotid TIA with distinct focal neurological dysfunction persisting <24 h, non-disabling stroke with a modified Rankin scale <3 and symptoms <24 h, or amaurosis fugax within previous 6 mo; results stratified by presence of contralateral carotid occlusion	CCO/No CCO (propensity matched cohort) Mean age: 69/69 y White: 91%/91% Female: 33%/34% DM: 38%/38% CAD (ischemic heart disease): 55%/55% COPD: NR HF: 17%/17% HTN: 91%/91% Smoker (history of): 80%/80% Stenosis: NR Prior contralateral CEA: NR Contralateral occlusion: 100%/0% Contralateral TIA/stroke: NR	High risk of selection bias and measurement bias; unclear how many procedures out of the total procedures done were included in the CARE registry and in this publication; unclear how much missing data they had; only 66% of patients got a post-procedure NIHSS assessment; unclear how outcomes were assessed for the other third of patients; not clear who was doing the assessments across sites, and how they were determining the presence of outcomes when not using NIHSS; in-hospital events only.	Poor
Rajamani, 2012[25]	Cohort study 1/2005-3/2011	CEA 4,149 (2,773)	CARE registry	Nationwide voluntary, hospital-based prospective database; results presented for adults age ≥70 y and stratified by age (70-74 and ≥75)	Overall Mean age: 78 y White: 96% Female: 41% DM: 32% CAD: NR COPD: 19% HF: NR HTN: 90% Smoker: 65% Stenosis: NR Prior contralateral CEA: NR Contralateral occlusion: NR Contralateral TIA/stroke: NR	High risk of selection bias and measurement bias; unclear how many procedures out of the total procedures done were included in the CARE registry and in this publication; unclear how much missing data they had; unclear how outcomes were assessed (encouraged use of NIHSS, but unclear how often it was used); not clear who was doing the assessments across sites, and how they were determining the presence of outcomes when not using NIHSS; in-hospital events only.	Poor
McKinlay, 2003[26], McKinlay, 2005[27], Zarins, 2009[28]	Non-randomized trial (CARESS) 4/2001-12/2002	CEA + CAAS 254 (170) CEA 254 (170) CAAS 143 (99)	Multicenter (14 sites), designed to evaluate the safety and effectiveness of CAAS with embolic protection compared with CEA. Choice of CAS/CEA was based on physician and patient preference.	Study designed to include a broad-risk population. Asymptomatic status was based on lack of symptoms associated with TIA or stroke in preceding 6 months. Only asymptomatic patients with ≥75% stenosis were included.	Mean age: 71 y White: 93% Female: 39% DM: 27% CAD: 64% COPD: NR HF: 15% HTN: 81% Smoker: NR Stenosis: 92% with >75% occlusion; 9% with 50%-75% Prior contralateral CEA: NR Contralateral occlusion: NR Contralateral TIA/stroke: NR	Unclear whether cases are representative of the source population, 46% of the cohort met at least one CMS-defined criteria of high risk for surgery (based on age or comorbidity). Participating principal investigators had to demonstrate a history of low complication rate with CEA or CAAS to participate.	Poor

Appendix E Table 2. Characteristics of Additional Studies Rated as Poor Quality and Reporting Rates of Periprocedural Complications of CEA or CAAS for Adults With Asymptomatic CAS

Data are for followup years, reported ages are the mean unless otherwise specified.

[a] Sample characteristics are of entire cohort (symptomatic and asymptomatic patients) unless otherwise noted.
[b] National Surgery Quality Improvement Program.
[c] Characteristics averaged across two time-periods.
[d] Study characteristics are a crude average of groups with and without life-limiting conditions. Those with life-limiting conditions were slightly older and had a higher incidence of diabetes, CAD, and HTN.
[e] Characteristics were given only for the total sample undergoing CAAS (symptomatic and asymptomatic patients). No patient characteristics were given for patients undergoing CEA.

Abbreviations: CCO = contralateral carotid artery occlusion; CEA = carotid endarterectomy; COPD = chronic obstructive pulmonary disease; CV = cerebrovascular; HF = heart failure; HTN = hypertension; N = sample size; U/S = ultrasound.

Appendix E Table 3. Results From Additional Studies Rated as Poor Quality and Reporting Rates of Periprocedural Complications of CEA or CAAS for Adults With Asymptomatic CAS

Study, Year	Method of Outcome Assessment	In-Hospital Rates	30-Day Rates
Horner, 2002[10]	Trained nurse reviewers, data reviewed/ edited by coordinating center; 30-day post-surgery questionnaire regarding health status and outcomes; clinical outcomes confirmed by medical record review.	NR	Stroke or death: Black: 2.1% Hispanic: 2.2% White: 1.6% Stroke, MI, or death: Black: 2.1% Hispanic: 3.2% White: 2.3% Any complication of the surgery: Black: 2.1% Hispanic :9.7% White: 5.5% Postoperative stay of 3 or more days: Black: 49.2% Hispanic: 52.2% White: 40.3% Return to the OR within 30 days: Black: 17.1% Hispanic: 12.9% White: 12.2% 1 or more returns to the OR related to CEA: Black: 9.3% Hispanic: 6.5% White: 3.1%
Samsa, 2002[11]	Trained nurse reviewers, ICD-9 codes, hospital-based followup included daily rounding, attending conferences, interviewing house staff, and the nurse epidemiologist regarding possible nosocomial infections and other complications. Reviewer called the patient at day 30 and interviewed patient or family member.	NR	30-day death, CVA, MI: Overall: 2.4% 1994-1995: 2.7% 1996-1997: 2.2% Variation across facility, 1994-1995: 0% to 9.5% Variation across facility, 1996-1997: 1.7% to 3.6%
Woo, 2010[12]	NSQIP uses Trained Surgical Clinical Reviewers at each site; independent chart review for identifying post-discharge morbidity	NR	Combined stroke and death: 1.4% Combined stroke, death and MI: 1.6% Stroke: 0.96% Death: 0.56% MI: 0.22% Peripheral nerve injury: 0.32% Wound infection: 0.68% Pneumonia: 0.66%
Garg, 201113	NSQIP uses Trained Surgical Clinical Reviewers at each site; independent chart review for identifying post-discharge morbidity	NR	Mortality: <1% Combined stroke/mortality: 1% Combined stroke/mortality/MI: 2%[a] Return to the OR within 30 days: 5% Unplanned intubation: 1.0% On ventilator >48 hours: 5%

Appendix E Table 3. Results From Additional Studies Rated as Poor Quality and Reporting Rates of Periprocedural Complications of CEA or CAAS for Adults With Asymptomatic CAS

Study, Year	Method of Outcome Assessment	In-Hospital Rates	30-Day Rates
Wallaert, 2012[14]	NSQIP uses Trained Surgical Clinical Reviewers at each site; independent chart review for identifying post-discharge morbidity	NR	Stroke or death: 1.4% Stroke or death for those >80: 2.2% Stroke or death in those with life-limiting conditions: 2.9% Stroke or death in those without life-limiting conditions: 1.1% Death in those with life-limiting conditions: 1.4% Death in those without life-limiting conditions: 0.3% Stroke in those with life-limiting conditions: 1.8% Stroke in those without life-limiting conditions: 0.9% 20% of CEAs performed in patients with at least one life-limiting condition 3% of CEAs performed in patients who had >1 life limiting condition
Theiss, 2008[16]	CND	Stroke or death: 2.7%	NR
Palombo, 2009[17]	NR	NR	Perioperative stroke: 0.8%
Micari, 2010[18]	30-day exam by independent neurologist	Major stroke: 0.08% Minor stroke: 0.08%	Combined death/stroke: 1.6%
Menyhei, 2011[19]	Each contributing country entered and validated its own data.	Stroke: 1.67%	Mortality: 0.38%
Lindstrom, 2012[20]	Deaths retrieved from Swedish National Population Registry; unclear for stroke (other than it is clear that they obtained the data from the registry, but not clear what exactly gets into the registry)	NR	Stroke or death: CAAS: 7.1% CEA: 4.0%
Sidawy, 2009[21]	CND	NR	CAAS: Combined death/stroke/MI: 4.60% Death: 1.99% Stroke: 2.11% MI: 1.37% TIA: 1.24% TMB/amaurosis fugax: 0.25% CEA: Combined death/stroke/MI: 1.97% Death: 0.70% Stroke: 1.28% MI: 0.58% TIA: 0.46% TMB/amaurosis fugax: 0.00%

Appendix E Table 3. Results From Additional Studies Rated as Poor Quality and Reporting Rates of Periprocedural Complications of CEA or CAAS for Adults With Asymptomatic CAS

Study, Year	Method of Outcome Assessment	In-Hospital Rates	30-Day Rates
Jim, 2012[23]	CND	NR	<65 CEA: Death: 0.79% Stroke: 1.31% MI: 0.39% Death/Stroke/MI: 2.10% <65 CAS: Death: 1.4% Stroke: 2.34% MI: 1.17% Death/Stroke/MI: 4.44% ≥65 CEA: Death: 0.72% Stroke: 1.81% MI: 1.20% Death/Stroke/MI: 3.31% ≥65 CAS: Death: 1.62% Stroke: 3.45% MI: 1.05% Death/Stroke/MI: 5.27%
Fokkema, 2013[15]	NSQIP uses Trained Surgical Clinical Reviewers at each site; independent chart review for identifying post-discharge morbidity	Stroke: 0.7% Death: 0.2% Cardiac event: 0.6% Combined stroke/death: 0.9% Combined stroke/death/cardiac event: 1.3%	Stroke: 1.1% Death: 0.5% Cardiac event: 0.8% Combined stroke/death: 1.5% Combined stroke/death/cardiac event: 2.1%
Schermerhorn, 2013[22]	CND	NR	High risk[b] CEA: Death: 1.3% Stroke: 2.7% MI: 1.6% Death/stroke: 3.7% Death/stroke/MI: 5.0% Non-high risk CEA: Death: 0.5% Stroke: 1.1% MI: 1.1% Death/stroke: 1.4% Death/stroke/MI: 2.2% High risk CAAS: Death: 1.7% Stroke: 3.4% MI: 1.1% Death/stroke: 4.8% Death/stroke/MI: 5.4% Non-high risk CAAS: Death: 1.6% Stroke: 2.6% MI: 1.0% Death/stroke: 3.6% Death/stroke/MI: 4.2%
Mercado, 2013[24]	Data are collected from existing medical records using standardized definitions, collection protocols, and tools. An on-site registry manager is designated by each participating center to ensure accuracy and timely submission.	CCO: Death/stroke/MI: 1.0% No CCO: Death/stroke/MI: 1.9%	NR

Appendix E Table 3. Results From Additional Studies Rated as Poor Quality and Reporting Rates of Periprocedural Complications of CEA or CAAS for Adults With Asymptomatic CAS

Study, Year	Method of Outcome Assessment	In-Hospital Rates	30-Day Rates
Rajamani, 2012[25]	Data are collected from existing medical records using standardized definitions, collection protocols, and tools. An on-site registry manager is designated by each participating center to ensure accuracy and timely submission.	Total: Death:0.5% Stroke:1.7% MI: 0.9% Death/stroke: 2.0% Death/stroke/MI: 2.7% Age 70-74 y: Death: 0.0% Stroke: 1.6% MI: 0.5% Death/stroke: 1.6% Death/stroke/MI: 2.0% Age >74 y: Death: 0.7% Stroke: 1.8% MI: 1.0% Death/stroke: 2.2% Death/stroke/MI: 3.1%	NR
McKinlay, 2003 (CaRESS Steering Committee)[26]; McKinlay, 2005[27]; Zarins, 2009[28]	Neurological examination, including NIHSS assessment and cerebral events questionnaires administered at 30 days by a neurologist not involved with the procedure. Independent data and safety monitoring board reviewed centrally adjudicated clinical events.	NR	CEA: All-cause mortality: 0.0% Stroke: 1.8% MI: 1.2% Death/stroke: 1.8% Death/stroke/MI: 3.0% CAAS: All-cause mortality: 0.0% Stroke: 1.0% MI: 0.0% Death/stroke: 1.0% Death/stroke/MI: 1.0%

Data are for followup years; reported ages are the mean unless otherwise specified.

[a] Study also reported <1% of the following harms: wound disruption, superficial incisional infection, pneumonia, pulmonary embolism, acute renal failure, progressive renal failure, urinary tract infection, coma >24 hours, peripheral nerve injury, cardiac arrest requiring CPR, myocardial infarction, bleeding/ transfusion, graft/prosthesis/flap failure, deep vein thrombosis requiring therapy, sepsis and septic shock.
[b] High risk criteria per CMS: age >79 years, NYHA CHF class III/IV, LVEF <30%, unstable angina, recent myocardial infarction, restenosis, radical neck dissection, contralateral occlusion, prior radiation to neck, contralateral laryngeal nerve injury, high anatomic lesion.

Abbreviations: CCO = contralateral carotid artery occlusion; CEA = carotid endarterectomy; COPD = chronic obstructive pulmonary disease; CV = cerebrovascular; HF = heart failure; HTN = hypertension; N = sample size; U/S = ultrasound.

Appendix E. References

1. Nowak J, Jogestrand T. Duplex ultrasonography is an efficient diagnostic tool for the detection of moderate to severe internal carotid artery stenosis. Clin Physiol Funct Imaging. 2007 May;27(3):144-7. PMID: 17445064.
2. Jogestrand T, Lindqvist M, Nowak J. Diagnostic performance of duplex ultrasonography in the detection of high grade internal carotid artery stenosis. Eur J Vasc Endovasc Surg. 2002 Jun;23(6):510-8. PMID: 12093067.
3. Jahromi AS, Cina CS, Liu Y, et al. Sensitivity and specificity of color duplex ultrasound measurement in the estimation of internal carotid artery stenosis: a systematic review and meta-analysis. J Vasc Surg. 2005 Jun;41(6):962-72. PMID: 15944595.
4. Nederkoorn PJ, Graaf Y, Hunink M. Duplex ultrasound and magnetic resonance angiography compared with digital subtraction angiography in carotid artery stenosis: a systematic review (Structured abstract). Stroke. 2003;34(5):1324-31. PMID: DARE-12003000974.
5. Blakeley DD, Oddone EZ, Hasselblad V, et al. Noninvasive carotid artery testing. A meta-analytic review. Ann Intern Med. 1995;122(5):360-7.
6. Hwang CS, Liao KM, Lee JH, et al. Measurement of carotid stenosis: comparisons between duplex and different angiographic grading methods. J Neuroimaging. 2003 Apr;13(2):133-9. PMID: 12722495.
7. Wolff T, Guirguis-Blake J, Miller T, et al. Screening for Asymptomatic Carotid Artery Stenosis. Evidence Synthesis Number 50. AHRQ Publication No. 08-05102-EF-1. Agency for Healthcare Research and Quality, December 2007 Rockville, MD.
8. Wolff T, Guirguis-Blake J, Miller T, et al. Screening for carotid artery stenosis: an update of the evidence for the U.S. Preventive Services Task Force. Ann Intern Med. 2007 Dec 18;147(12):860-70. PMID: 18087057.
9. Sabeti S, Schillinger M, Mlekusch W, et al. Quantification of internal carotid artery stenosis with duplex US: comparative analysis of different flow velocity criteria. Radiology. 2004 Aug;232(2):431-9. PMID: 15286315.
10. Horner RD, Oddone EZ, Stechuchak KM, et al. Racial variations in postoperative outcomes of carotid endarterectomy: evidence from the Veterans Affairs National Surgical Quality Improvement Program. Med Care. 2002 Jan;40(1 Suppl):I35-43. PMID: 11789630.
11. Samsa G, Oddone EZ, Horner R, et al. To what extent should quality of care decisions be based on health outcomes data? Application to carotid endarterectomy. Stroke. 2002 Dec;33(12):2944-9. PMID: 12468795.
12. Woo K, Garg J, Hye RJ, et al. Contemporary results of carotid endarterectomy for asymptomatic carotid stenosis. Stroke. 2010 May;41(5):975-9. PMID: 20339122.
13. Garg J, Frankel DA, Dilley RB. Carotid endarterectomy in academic versus community hospitals: the national surgical quality improvement program data. Ann Vasc Surg. 2011 May;25(4):433-41. PMID: 21435832.
14. Wallaert JB, De Martino RR, Finlayson SR, et al. Carotid endarterectomy in asymptomatic patients with limited life expectancy. Stroke. 2012 Jul;43(7):1781-7. PMID: 22550053.
15. Fokkema M, Bensley RP, Lo RC, et al. In-hospital versus postdischarge adverse events following carotid endarterectomy. J Vasc Surg. 2013 Jun;57(6):1568-75, 75 e1-3. PMID: 23388394.
16. Theiss W, Hermanek P, Mathias K, et al. Predictors of death and stroke after carotid angioplasty and stenting: a subgroup analysis of the Pro-CAS data. Stroke. 2008 Aug;39(8):2325-30. PMID: 18583556.
17. Palombo D, Lucertini G, Mambrini S, et al. Carotid endarterectomy: results of the Italian Vascular Registry. J Cardiovasc Surg (Torino). 2009 Apr;50(2):183-7. PMID: 19282808.
18. Micari A, Stabile E, Cremonesi A, et al. Carotid artery stenting in octogenarians using a proximal endovascular occlusion cerebral protection device: a multicenter registry. Catheter Cardiovasc Interv. 2010 Jul 1;76(1):9-15. PMID: 20578188.
19. Menyhei G, Bjorck M, Beiles B, et al. Outcome following carotid endarterectomy: lessons learned from a large international vascular registry. Eur J Vasc Endovasc Surg. 2011 Jun;41(6):735-40. PMID: 21450496.
20. Lindstrom D, Jonsson M, Formgren J, et al. Outcome after 7 years of carotid artery stenting and endarterectomy in Sweden - single centre and national results. Eur J Vasc Endovasc Surg. 2012 May;43(5):499-503. PMID: 22342694.
21. Sidawy AN, Zwolak RM, White RA, et al. Risk-adjusted 30-day outcomes of carotid stenting and endarterectomy: results from the SVS Vascular Registry. J Vasc Surg. 2009 Jan;49(1):71-9. PMID: 19028045.
22. Schermerhorn ML, Fokkema M, Goodney P, et al. The impact of Centers for Medicare and Medicaid Services high-risk criteria on outcome after carotid endarterectomy and carotid artery stenting in the SVS Vascular Registry. J Vasc Surg. 2013 May;57(5):1318-24. PMID: 23406712.
23. Jim J, Rubin BG, Ricotta JJ, 2nd, et al. Society for Vascular Surgery (SVS) Vascular Registry evaluation of comparative effectiveness of carotid revascularization procedures stratified by Medicare age. J Vasc Surg. 2012 May;55(5):1313-20; discussion 21. PMID: 22459755.

Appendix E. References

24. Mercado N, Cohen DJ, Spertus JA, et al. Carotid artery stenting of a contralateral occlusion and in-hospital outcomes: results from the CARE (Carotid Artery Revascularization and Endarterectomy) registry. JACC Cardiovasc Interv. 2013 Jan;6(1):59-64. PMID: 23347862.

25. Rajamani K, Kennedy KF, Ruggiero NJ, et al. Outcomes of carotid endarterctomy in the elderly: A report from the care registry(registered trademark). Stroke. 2012;43(2).

26. CaRESS Steering Committee. Carotid revascularization using endarterectomy or stenting systems (CARESS): Phase I clinical trial. J Endovasc Ther. 2003 Dec;10(6):1021-30. PMID: 14723574.

27. McKinlay SM. Carotid Revascularization Using Endarterectomy or Stenting Systems (CaRESS) phase I clinical trial: 1-Year results. J Vasc Surg. 2005;42(2):213-9.

28. Zarins CK, White RA, Diethrich EB, et al. Carotid revascularization using endarterectomy or stenting systems (CaRESS): 4-year outcomes. J Endovasc Ther. 2009 Aug;16(4):397-409. PMID: 19702339.

Appendix F Figure 1. Ipsilateral Stroke (Nonperioperative) for CEA Compared With Medical Therapy

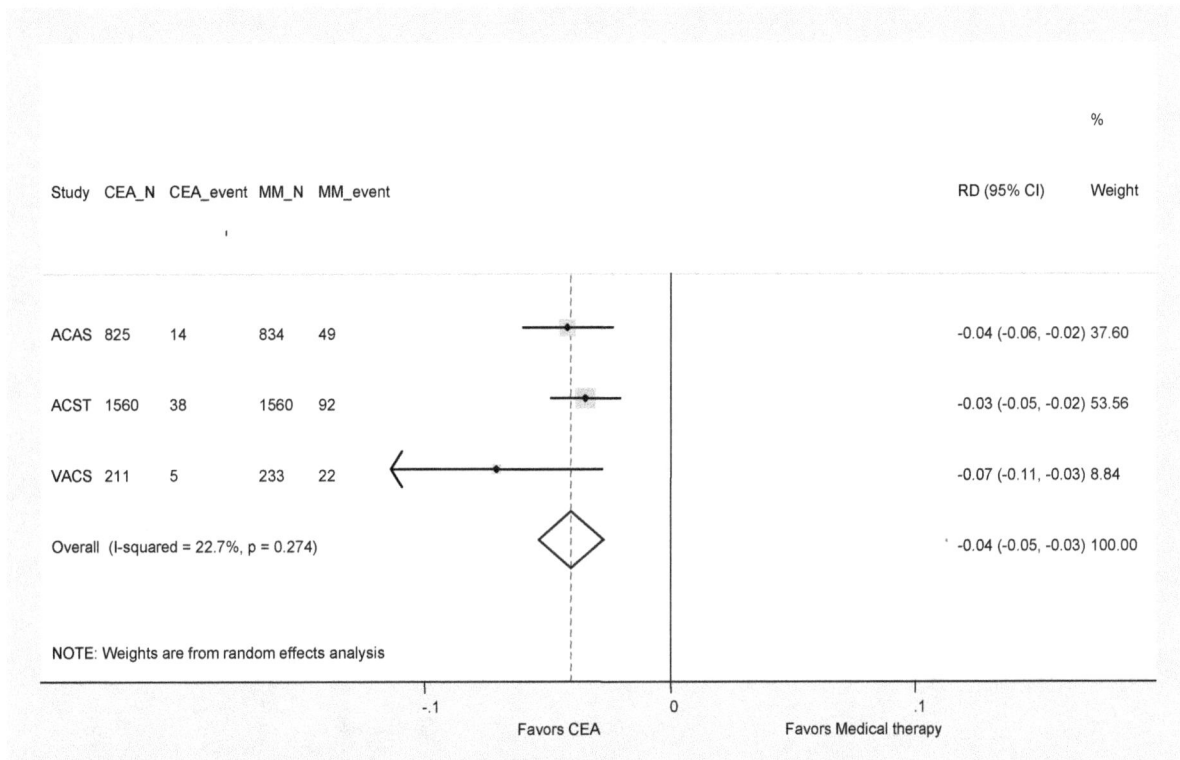

Study	RD	[95% Conf. Interval]		% Weight
ACAS	-0.042	-0.060	-0.024	37.60
ACST	-0.035	-0.049	-0.021	53.56
VACS	-0.071	-0.114	-0.028	8.84
D+L pooled RD	-0.041	-0.054	-0.027	100.00

Appendix F Figure 2. Any Stroke (Nonperioperative) for CEA Compared With Medical Therapy

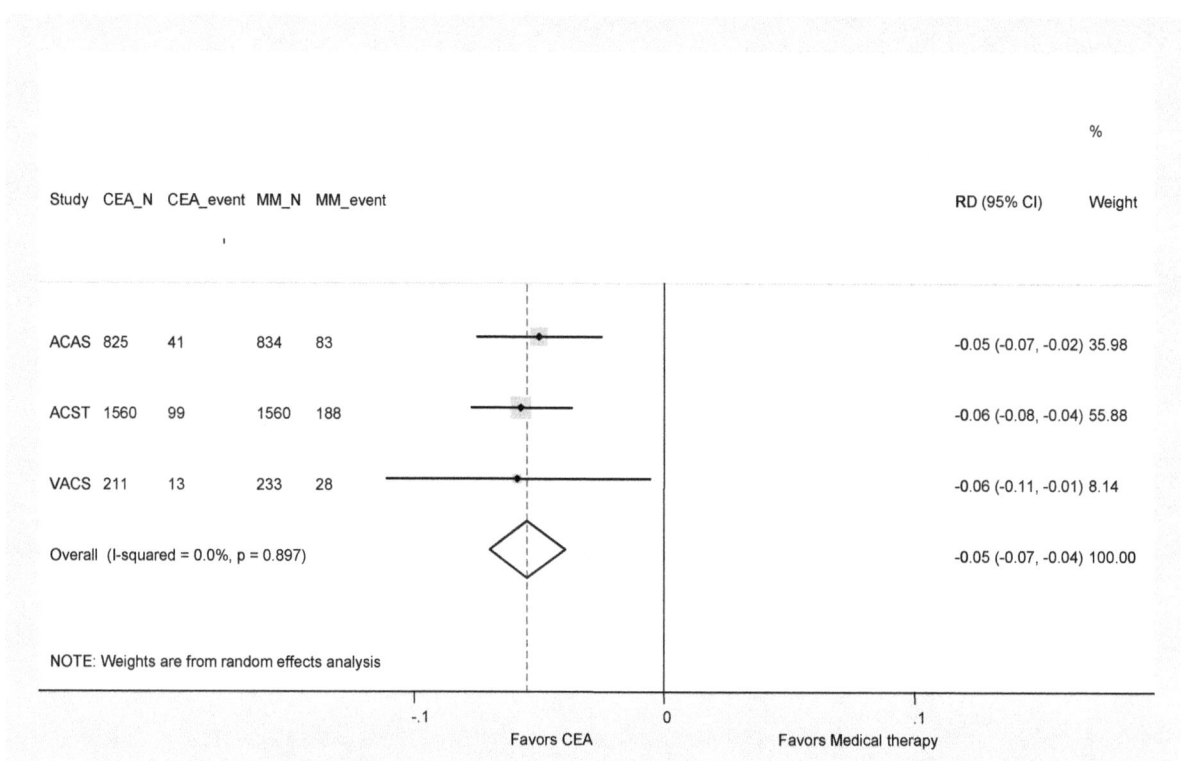

Study	RD	[95% Conf. Interval]		% Weight
ACAS	-0.050	-0.075	-0.025	35.98
ACST	-0.057	-0.077	-0.037	55.88
VACS	-0.059	-0.111	-0.006	8.14
D+L pooled RD	-0.055	-0.070	-0.039	100.00

Appendix F Figure 3. Perioperative Stroke/Death or Any Subsequent Stroke for CEA Compared With Medical Therapy

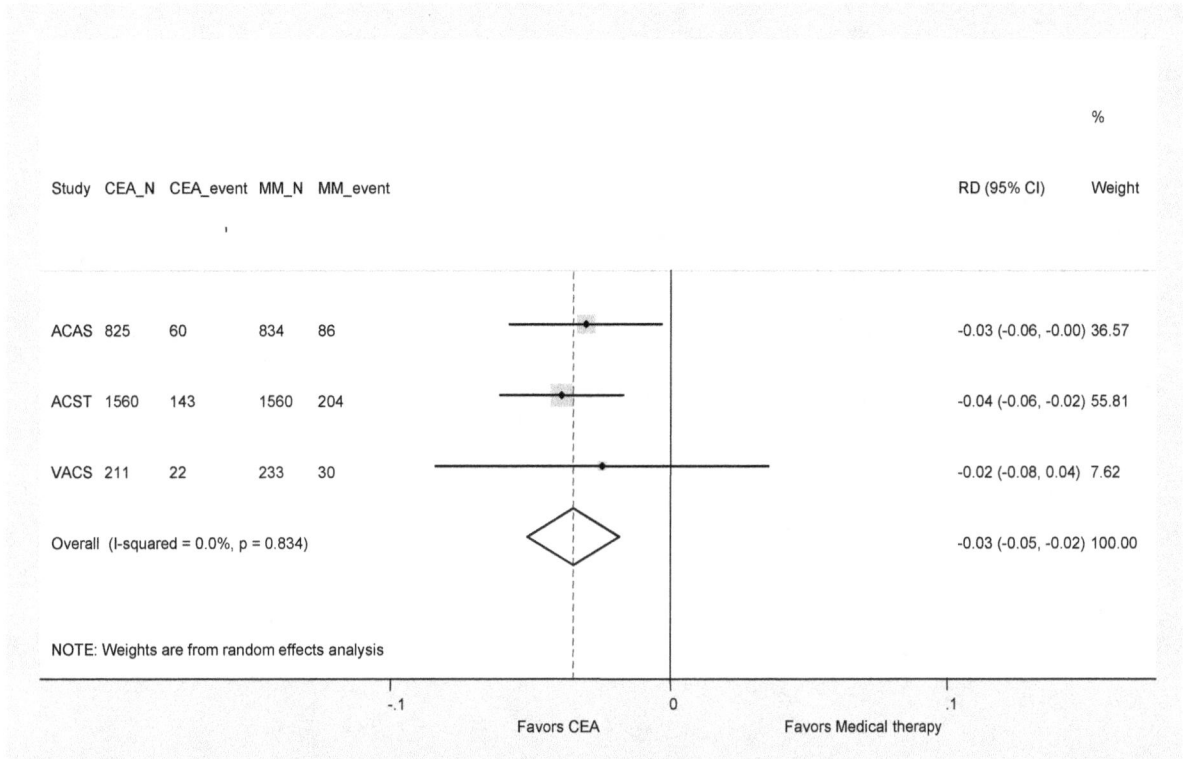

Study	CEA_N	CEA_event	MM_N	MM_event	RD (95% CI)	% Weight
ACAS	825	60	834	86	-0.03 (-0.06, -0.00)	36.57
ACST	1560	143	1560	204	-0.04 (-0.06, -0.02)	55.81
VACS	211	22	233	30	-0.02 (-0.08, 0.04)	7.62
Overall (I-squared = 0.0%, p = 0.834)					-0.03 (-0.05, -0.02)	100.00

NOTE: Weights are from random effects analysis

Favors CEA — Favors Medical therapy

Study	RD	[95% Conf. Interval]		% Weight
ACAS	-0.030	-0.058	-0.003	36.57
ACST	-0.039	-0.061	-0.017	55.81
VACS	-0.024	-0.084	0.035	7.62
D+L pooled RD	-0.035	-0.051	-0.018	100.00

Appendix F Figure 4. Perioperative Stroke/Death or Any Subsequent Stroke for CEA Compared With Medical Therapy, Sensitivity Analysis Including Angiogram-Related Events

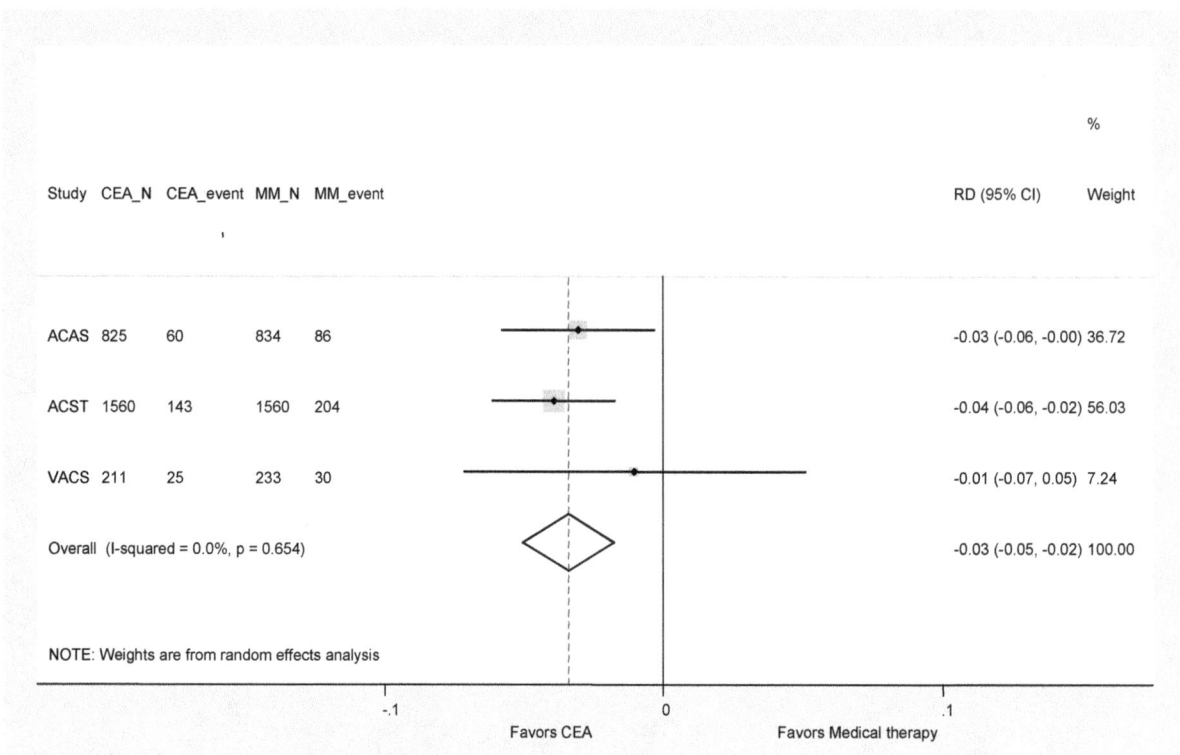

Study	CEA_N	CEA_event	MM_N	MM_event		RD (95% CI)	% Weight
ACAS	825	60	834	86		-0.03 (-0.06, -0.00)	36.72
ACST	1560	143	1560	204		-0.04 (-0.06, -0.02)	56.03
VACS	211	25	233	30		-0.01 (-0.07, 0.05)	7.24
Overall (I-squared = 0.0%, p = 0.654)						-0.03 (-0.05, -0.02)	100.00

NOTE: Weights are from random effects analysis

Favors CEA — Favors Medical therapy

```
       Study    |   RD    [95% Conf. Interval]    % Weight
----------------+---------------------------------------------
ACAS            | -0.030   -0.058   -0.003        36.72
ACST            | -0.039   -0.061   -0.017        56.03
VACS            | -0.010   -0.072    0.051         7.24
----------------+---------------------------------------------
D+L pooled RD   | -0.034   -0.050   -0.017        100.00
----------------+---------------------------------------------
```

Appendix F Figure 5. Perioperative Stroke/Death or Any Subsequent Ipsilateral Stroke for CEA Compared With Medical Therapy

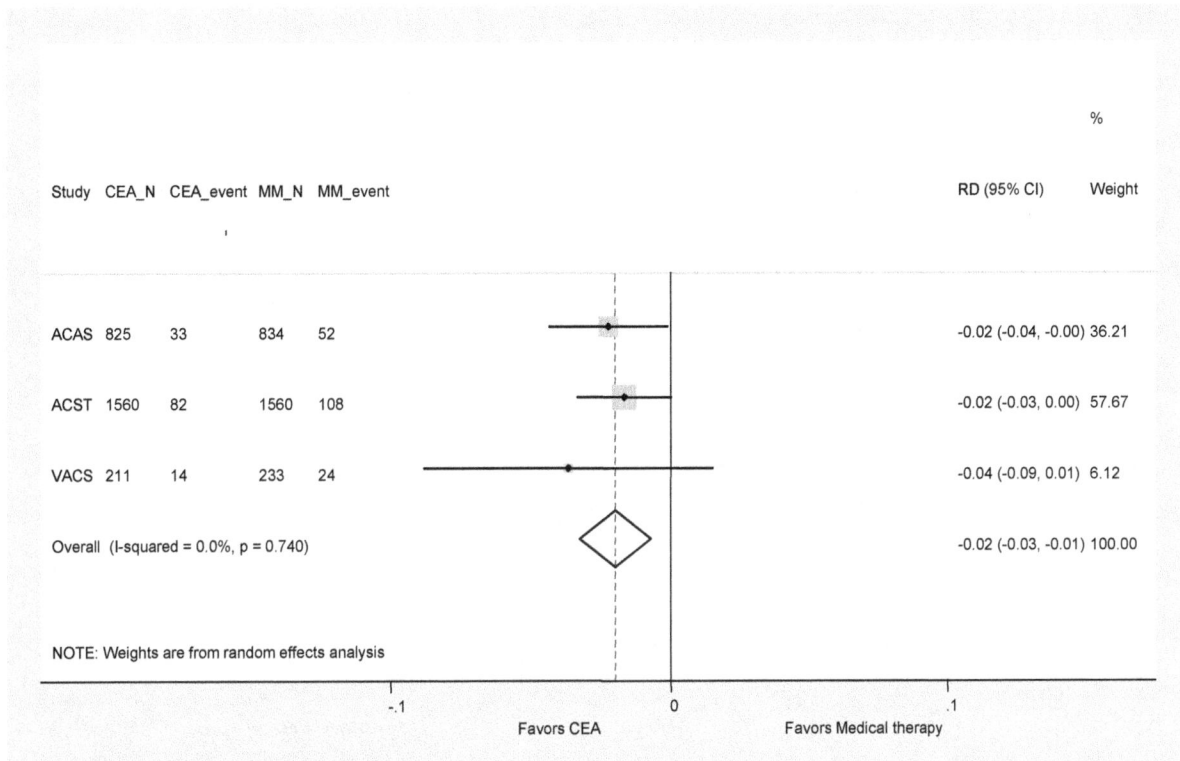

Study	RD	[95% Conf. Interval]		% Weight
ACAS	-0.022	-0.044	-0.001	36.21
ACST	-0.017	-0.033	0.000	57.67
VACS	-0.037	-0.088	0.015	6.12
D+L pooled RD	-0.020	-0.033	-0.007	100.00

Appendix F Figure 6. Perioperative Stroke/Death or Any Subsequent Ipsilateral Stroke for CEA Compared With Medical Therapy, Sensitivity Analysis Including Angiogram-Related Events

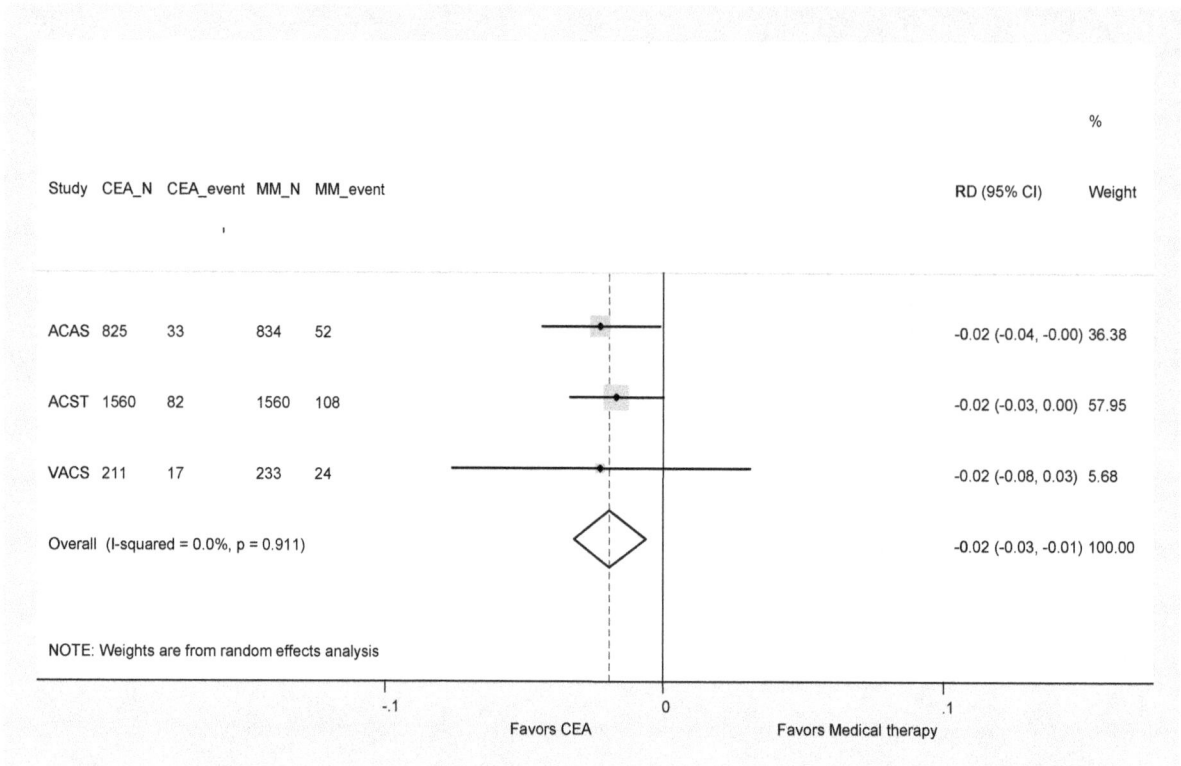

Study	CEA_N	CEA_event	MM_N	MM_event	RD (95% CI)	% Weight
ACAS	825	33	834	52	-0.02 (-0.04, -0.00)	36.38
ACST	1560	82	1560	108	-0.02 (-0.03, 0.00)	57.95
VACS	211	17	233	24	-0.02 (-0.08, 0.03)	5.68
Overall (I-squared = 0.0%, p = 0.911)					-0.02 (-0.03, -0.01)	100.00

NOTE: Weights are from random effects analysis

Favors CEA — Favors Medical therapy

```
        Study    |   RD    [95% Conf. Interval]   % Weight
-----------------+------------------------------------------
ACAS             | -0.022   -0.044   -0.001        36.38
ACST             | -0.017   -0.033    0.000        57.95
VACS             | -0.022   -0.076    0.031         5.68
-----------------+------------------------------------------
D+L pooled RD    | -0.019   -0.032   -0.006       100.00
-----------------+------------------------------------------
```

Appendix F Figure 7. All-Cause Mortality for CEA Compared With Medical Therapy

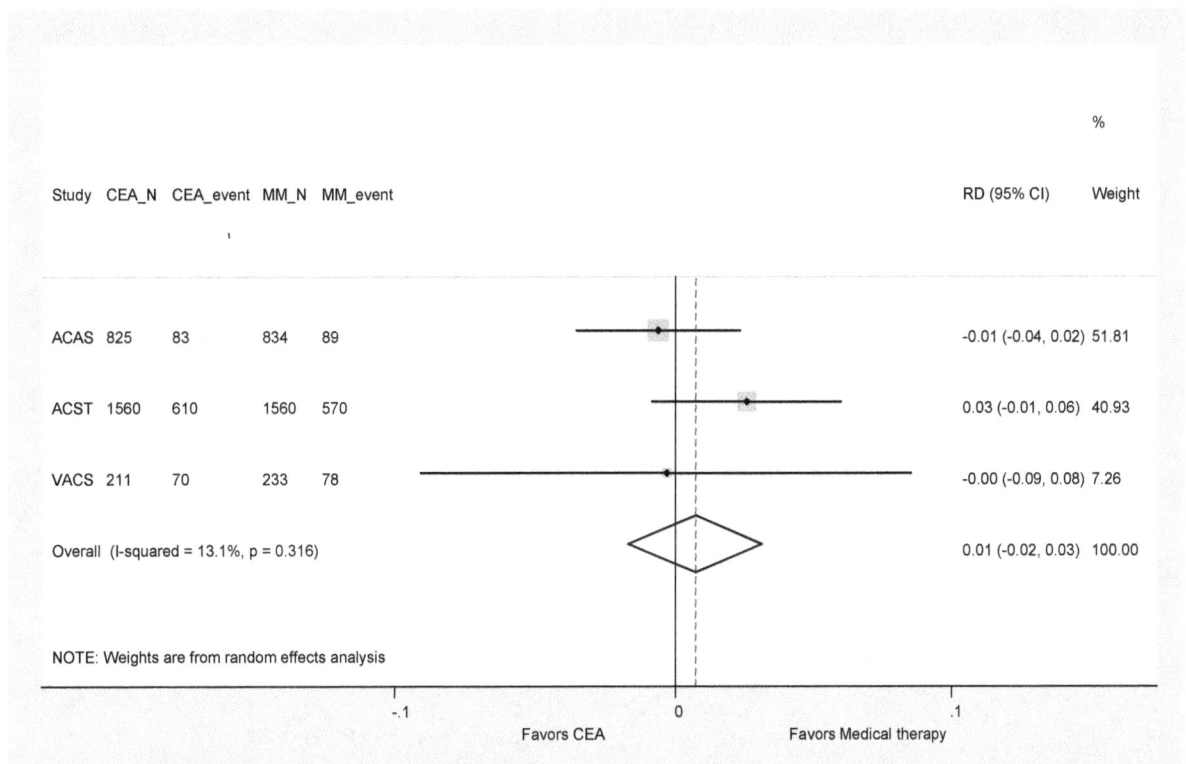

Study	RD	[95% Conf. Interval]		% Weight
ACAS	-0.006	-0.035	0.023	51.81
ACST	0.026	-0.008	0.060	40.93
VACS	-0.003	-0.091	0.085	7.26
D+L pooled RD	0.007	-0.017	0.031	100.00

Appendix F Figure 8. Any Stroke or Death for CEA Compared With Medical Therapy

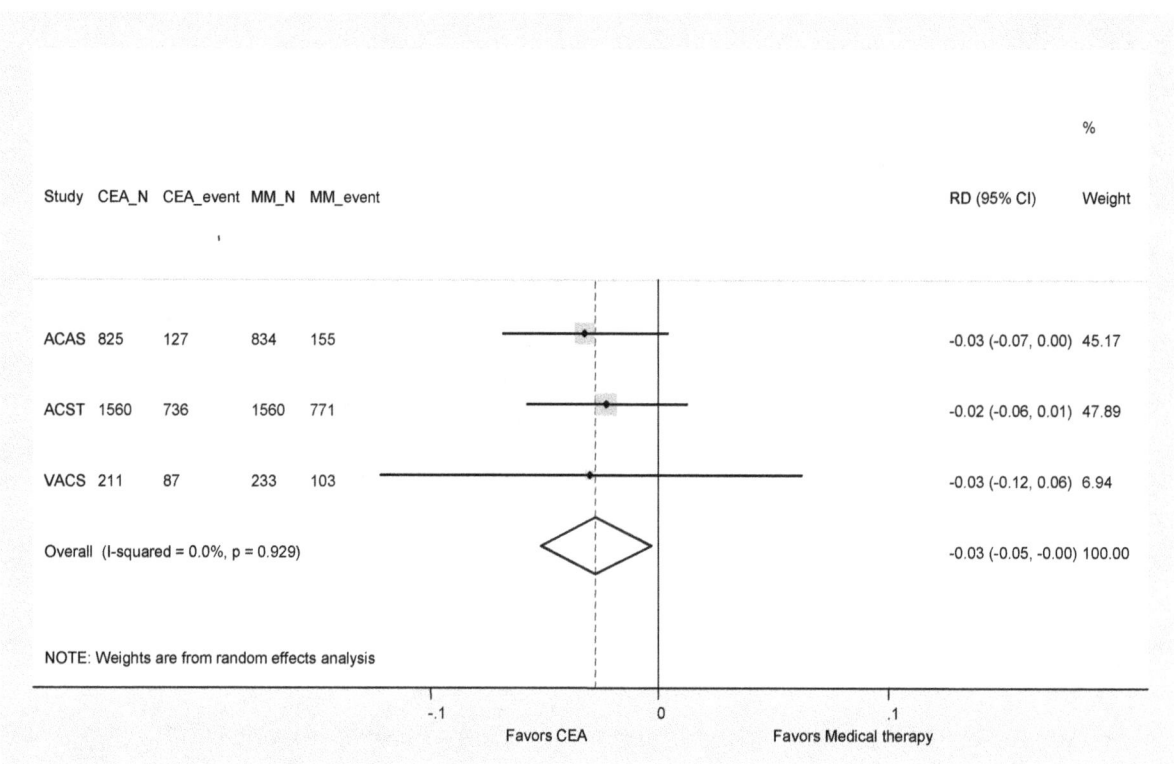

Study	CEA_N	CEA_event	MM_N	MM_event	RD (95% CI)	% Weight
ACAS	825	127	834	155	-0.03 (-0.07, 0.00)	45.17
ACST	1560	736	1560	771	-0.02 (-0.06, 0.01)	47.89
VACS	211	87	233	103	-0.03 (-0.12, 0.06)	6.94
Overall (I-squared = 0.0%, p = 0.929)					-0.03 (-0.05, -0.00)	100.00

NOTE: Weights are from random effects analysis

Favors CEA   Favors Medical therapy

```
        Study   |   RD    [95% Conf. Interval]   % Weight
----------------+------------------------------------------
          ACAS  | -0.032   -0.068    0.004        45.17
          ACST  | -0.022   -0.057    0.013        47.89
          VACS  | -0.030   -0.122    0.062         6.94
----------------+------------------------------------------
  D+L pooled RD | -0.027   -0.051   -0.003       100.00
----------------+------------------------------------------
```

Appendix F Figure 9. Perioperative Stroke or Death for CEA Compared With Medical Therapy

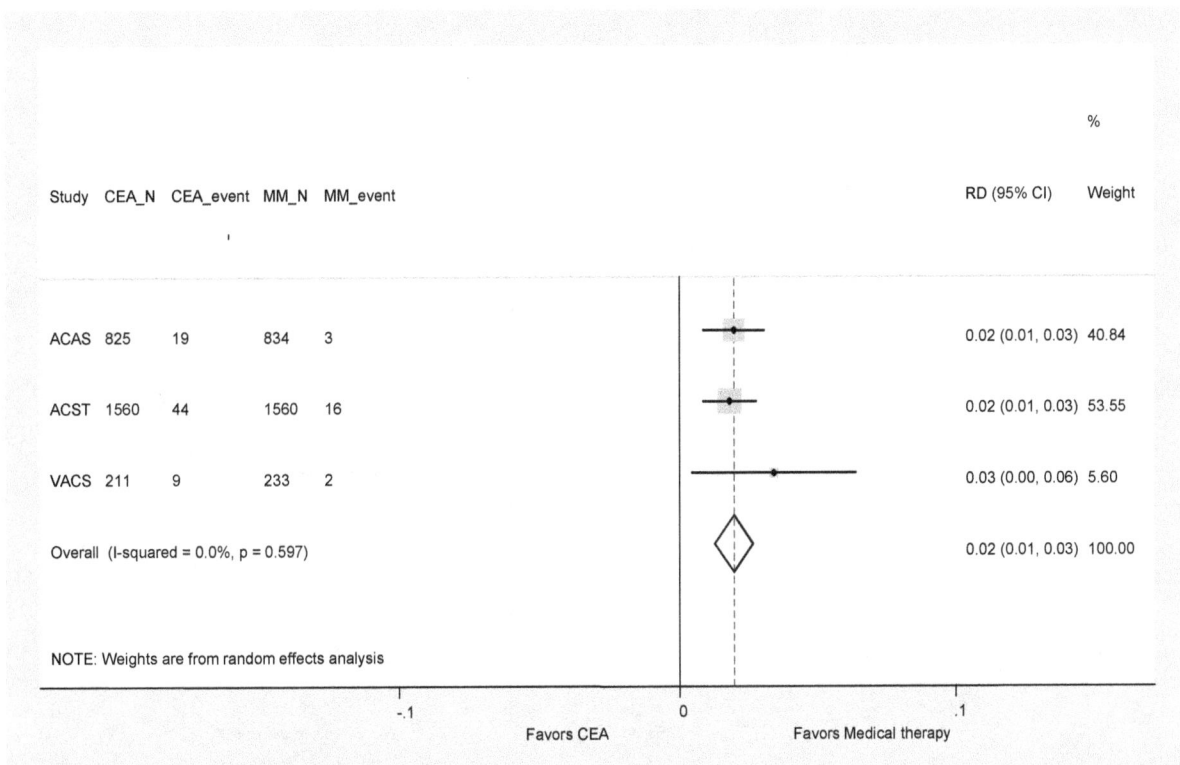

Study	RD	[95% Conf. Interval]		% Weight
ACAS	0.019	0.008	0.030	40.84
ACST	0.018	0.008	0.028	53.55
VACS	0.034	0.004	0.064	5.60
D+L pooled RD	0.019	0.012	0.026	100.00

Appendix F Figure 10. Perioperative Stroke or Death for CEA Compared With Medical Therapy, Sensitivity Analysis Including Angiogram-Related Events

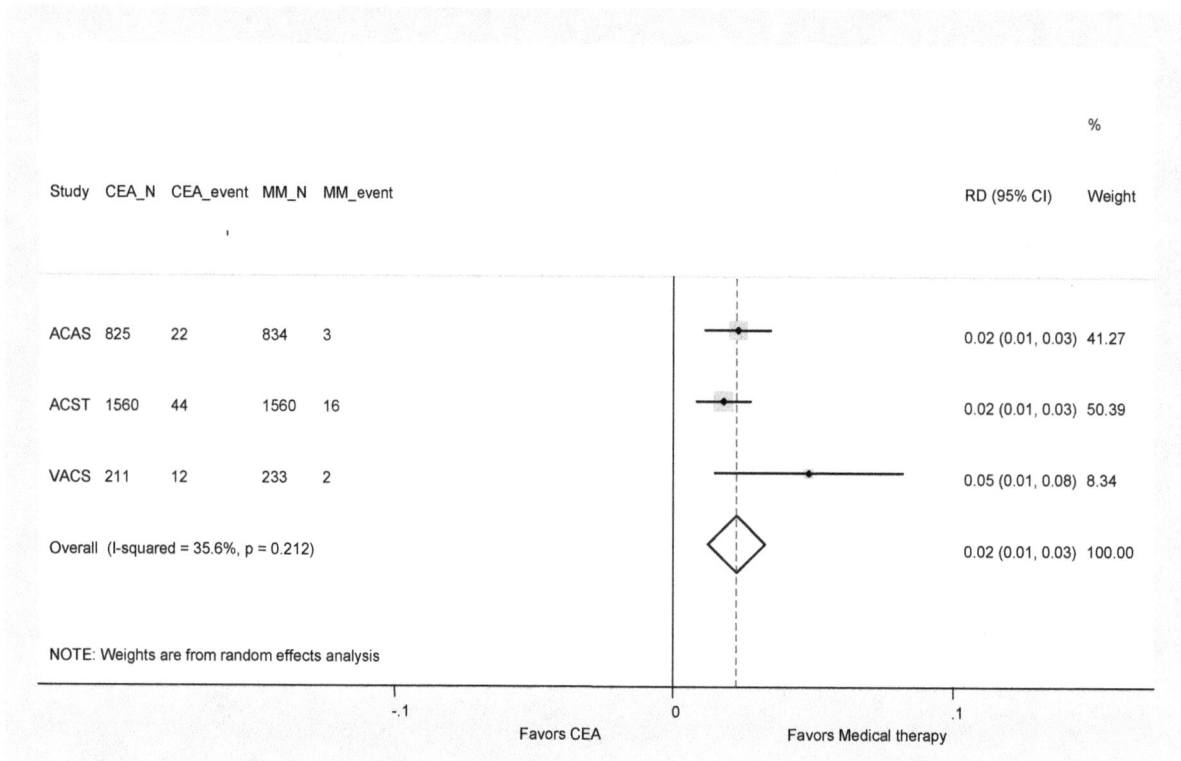

Study	CEA_N	CEA_event	MM_N	MM_event	RD (95% CI)	% Weight
ACAS	825	22	834	3	0.02 (0.01, 0.03)	41.27
ACST	1560	44	1560	16	0.02 (0.01, 0.03)	50.39
VACS	211	12	233	2	0.05 (0.01, 0.08)	8.34
Overall (I-squared = 35.6%, p = 0.212)					0.02 (0.01, 0.03)	100.00

NOTE: Weights are from random effects analysis

Favors CEA   Favors Medical therapy

```
   Study      |   RD    [95% Conf. Interval]   % Weight
--------------+-------------------------------------------
ACAS          |  0.023    0.011    0.035        41.27
ACST          |  0.018    0.008    0.028        50.39
VACS          |  0.048    0.015    0.082         8.34
--------------+-------------------------------------------
D+L pooled RD |  0.023    0.012    0.033       100.00
--------------+-------------------------------------------
```

Appendix F Figure 11. Perioperative Nonfatal Myocardial Infarction for CEA Compared With Medical Therapy

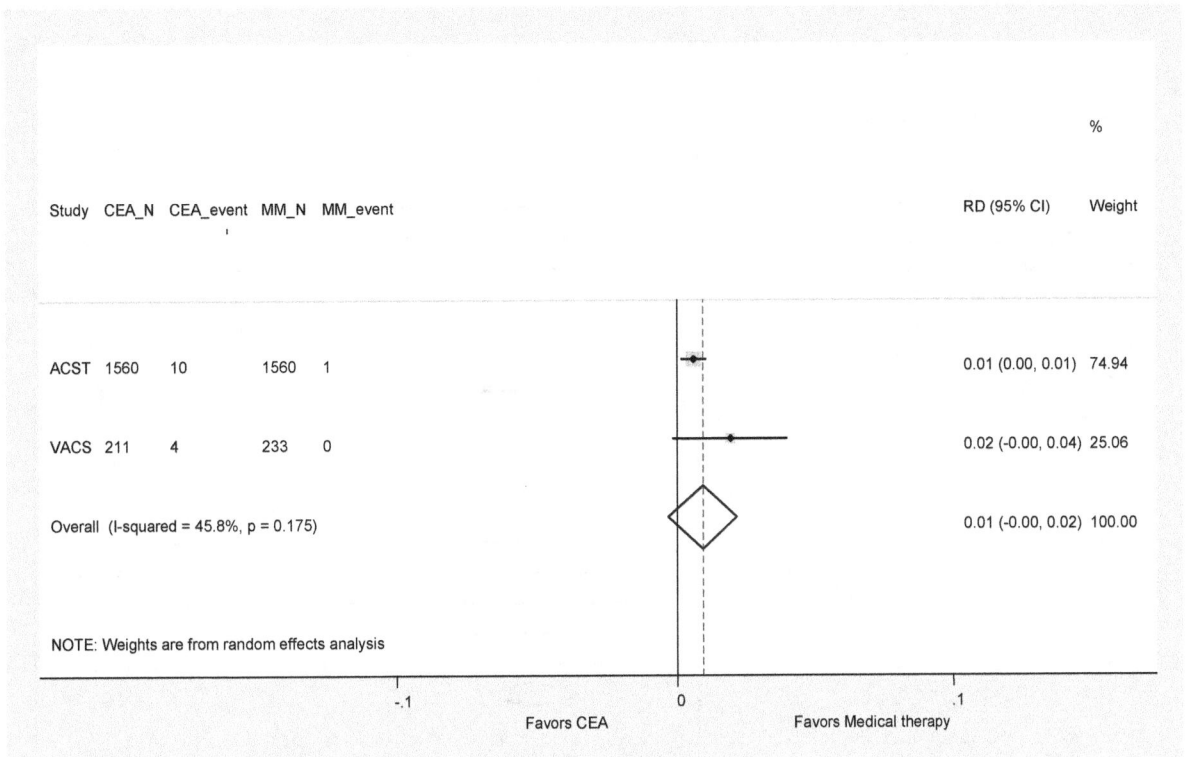

Study		RD	[95% Conf. Interval]		% Weight
ACST		0.006	0.002	0.010	74.94
VACS		0.019	-0.001	0.039	25.06
D+L pooled RD		0.009	-0.003	0.021	100.00

Appendix F Figure 12. Perioperative Death or Stroke Rate After CEA, by Study Design

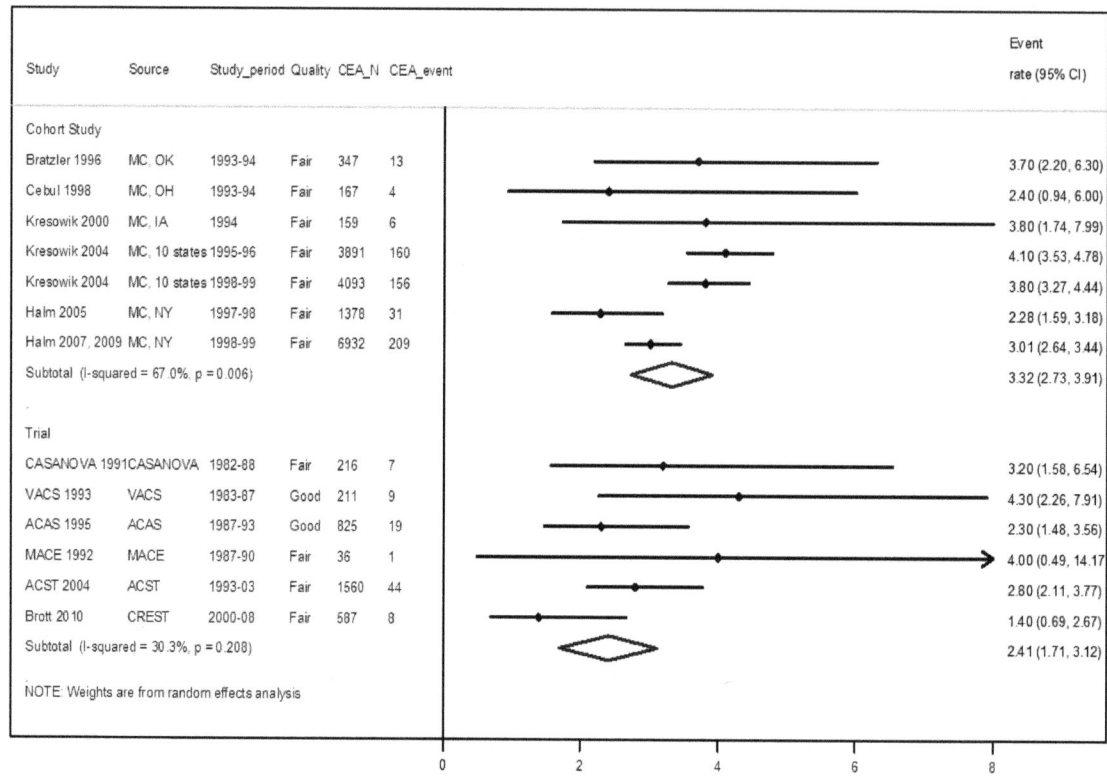

Study	Source	Study_period	Quality	CEA_N	CEA_event		Event rate (95% CI)
Cohort Study							
Bratzler 1996	MC, OK	1993-94	Fair	347	13		3.70 (2.20, 6.30)
Cebul 1998	MC, OH	1993-94	Fair	167	4		2.40 (0.94, 6.00)
Kresowik 2000	MC, IA	1994	Fair	159	6		3.80 (1.74, 7.99)
Kresowik 2004	MC, 10 states	1995-96	Fair	3891	160		4.10 (3.53, 4.78)
Kresowik 2004	MC, 10 states	1998-99	Fair	4093	156		3.80 (3.27, 4.44)
Halm 2005	MC, NY	1997-98	Fair	1378	31		2.28 (1.59, 3.18)
Halm 2007, 2009	MC, NY	1998-99	Fair	6932	209		3.01 (2.64, 3.44)
Subtotal (I-squared = 67.0%, p = 0.006)							3.32 (2.73, 3.91)
Trial							
CASANOVA 1991	CASANOVA	1982-88	Fair	216	7		3.20 (1.58, 6.54)
VACS 1993	VACS	1983-87	Good	211	9		4.30 (2.26, 7.91)
ACAS 1995	ACAS	1987-93	Good	825	19		2.30 (1.48, 3.56)
MACE 1992	MACE	1987-90	Fair	36	1		4.00 (0.49, 14.17)
ACST 2004	ACST	1993-03	Fair	1560	44		2.80 (2.11, 3.77)
Brott 2010	CREST	2000-08	Fair	587	8		1.40 (0.69, 2.67)
Subtotal (I-squared = 30.3%, p = 0.208)							2.41 (1.71, 3.12)

NOTE: Weights are from random effects analysis

Appendix F Figure 13. Perioperative Death or Stroke Rate After CEA, Sensitivity Analysis Including Studies Rated as Poor Quality, by Study Design

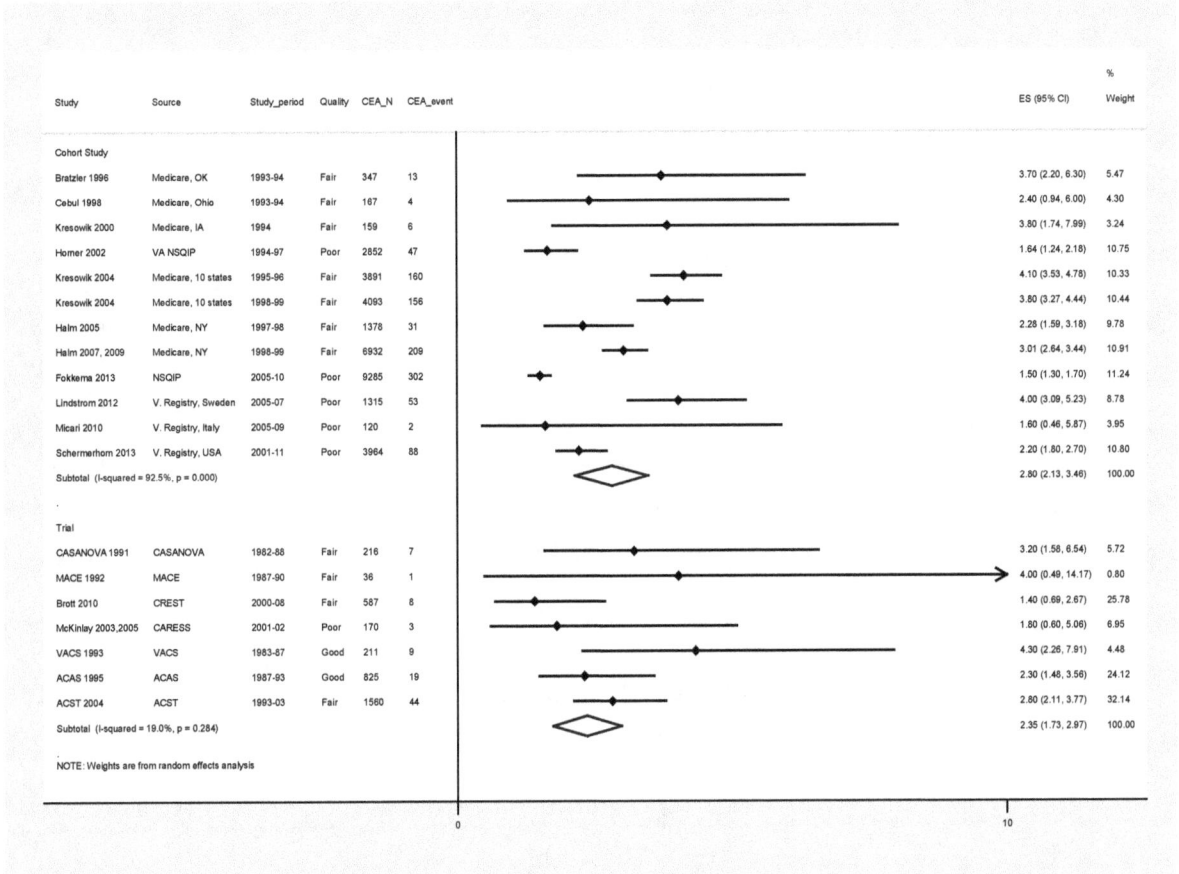

Study	Source	Study_period	Quality	CEA_N	CEA_event	ES (95% CI)	% Weight
Cohort Study							
Bratzler 1996	Medicare, OK	1993-94	Fair	347	13	3.70 (2.20, 6.30)	5.47
Cebul 1998	Medicare, Ohio	1993-94	Fair	167	4	2.40 (0.94, 6.00)	4.30
Kresowik 2000	Medicare, IA	1994	Fair	159	6	3.80 (1.74, 7.99)	3.24
Horner 2002	VA NSQIP	1994-97	Poor	2852	47	1.64 (1.24, 2.18)	10.75
Kresowik 2004	Medicare, 10 states	1995-96	Fair	3891	160	4.10 (3.53, 4.78)	10.33
Kresowik 2004	Medicare, 10 states	1998-99	Fair	4093	156	3.80 (3.27, 4.44)	10.44
Halm 2005	Medicare, NY	1997-98	Fair	1378	31	2.28 (1.59, 3.18)	9.78
Halm 2007, 2009	Medicare, NY	1998-99	Fair	6932	209	3.01 (2.64, 3.44)	10.91
Fokkema 2013	NSQIP	2005-10	Poor	9285	302	1.50 (1.30, 1.70)	11.24
Lindstrom 2012	V. Registry, Sweden	2005-07	Poor	1315	53	4.00 (3.09, 5.23)	8.78
Micari 2010	V. Registry, Italy	2005-09	Poor	120	2	1.60 (0.46, 5.87)	3.95
Schermerhorn 2013	V. Registry, USA	2001-11	Poor	3964	88	2.20 (1.80, 2.70)	10.80
Subtotal (I-squared = 92.5%, p = 0.000)						2.80 (2.13, 3.46)	100.00
Trial							
CASANOVA 1991	CASANOVA	1982-88	Fair	216	7	3.20 (1.58, 6.54)	5.72
MACE 1992	MACE	1987-90	Fair	36	1	4.00 (0.49, 14.17)	0.80
Brott 2010	CREST	2000-08	Fair	587	8	1.40 (0.69, 2.67)	25.78
McKinlay 2003, 2005	CARESS	2001-02	Poor	170	3	1.80 (0.60, 5.06)	6.95
VACS 1993	VACS	1983-87	Good	211	9	4.30 (2.26, 7.91)	4.48
ACAS 1995	ACAS	1987-93	Good	825	19	2.30 (1.48, 3.56)	24.12
ACST 2004	ACST	1993-03	Fair	1560	44	2.80 (2.11, 3.77)	32.14
Subtotal (I-squared = 19.0%, p = 0.284)						2.35 (1.73, 2.97)	100.00

NOTE: Weights are from random effects analysis

Appendix F Figure 14. Perioperative Death or Stroke Rate After CAAS, by Study Design

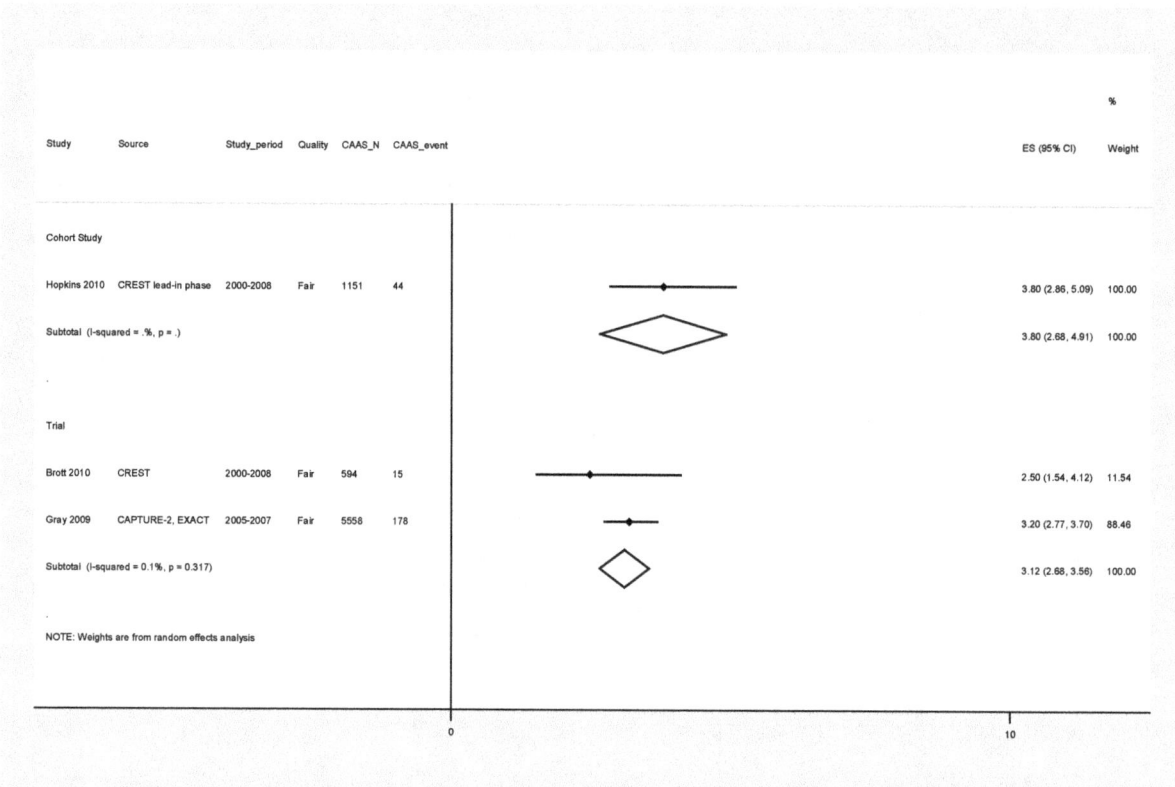

Study	Source	Study_period	Quality	CAAS_N	CAAS_event	ES (95% CI)	% Weight
Cohort Study							
Hopkins 2010	CREST lead-in phase	2000-2008	Fair	1151	44	3.80 (2.86, 5.09)	100.00
Subtotal (I-squared = .%, p = .)						3.80 (2.68, 4.91)	100.00
Trial							
Brott 2010	CREST	2000-2008	Fair	594	15	2.50 (1.54, 4.12)	11.54
Gray 2009	CAPTURE-2, EXACT	2005-2007	Fair	5558	178	3.20 (2.77, 3.70)	88.46
Subtotal (I-squared = 0.1%, p = 0.317)						3.12 (2.68, 3.56)	100.00

NOTE: Weights are from random effects analysis

0   10

Appendix F Figure 15. Perioperative Death or Stroke Rate After CAAS, Sensitivity Analysis Including Studies Rated as Poor Quality, by Study Design

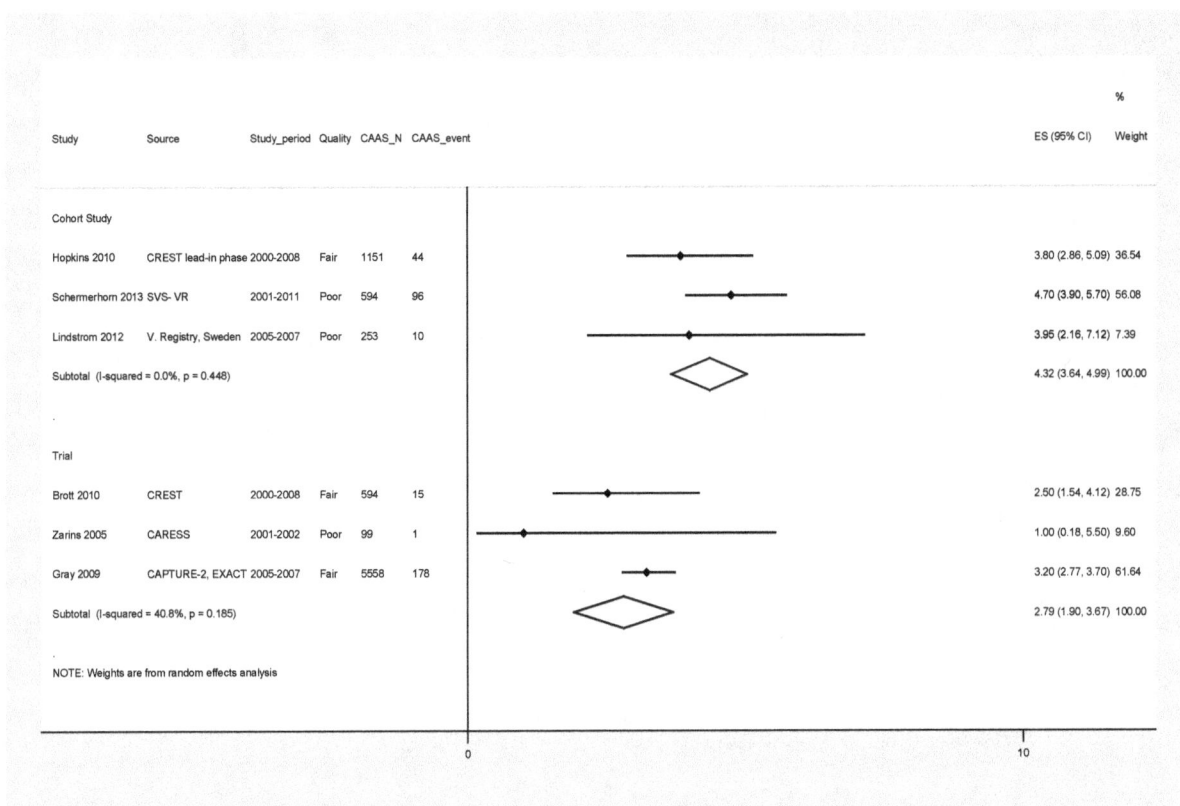

Study	Source	Study_period	Quality	CAAS_N	CAAS_event	ES (95% CI)	% Weight
Cohort Study							
Hopkins 2010	CREST lead-in phase	2000-2008	Fair	1151	44	3.80 (2.86, 5.09)	36.54
Schermerhorn 2013	SVS- VR	2001-2011	Poor	594	96	4.70 (3.90, 5.70)	56.08
Lindstrom 2012	V. Registry, Sweden	2005-2007	Poor	253	10	3.95 (2.16, 7.12)	7.39
Subtotal (I-squared = 0.0%, p = 0.448)						4.32 (3.64, 4.99)	100.00
Trial							
Brott 2010	CREST	2000-2008	Fair	594	15	2.50 (1.54, 4.12)	28.75
Zarins 2005	CARESS	2001-2002	Poor	99	1	1.00 (0.18, 5.50)	9.60
Gray 2009	CAPTURE-2, EXACT	2005-2007	Fair	5558	178	3.20 (2.77, 3.70)	61.64
Subtotal (I-squared = 40.8%, p = 0.185)						2.79 (1.90, 3.67)	100.00

NOTE: Weights are from random effects analysis

Appendix F Figure 16. Ipsilateral Stroke (Nonperioperative) for CEA Compared With Medical Therapy, Sensitivity Analysis Using Profile Likelihood Methods

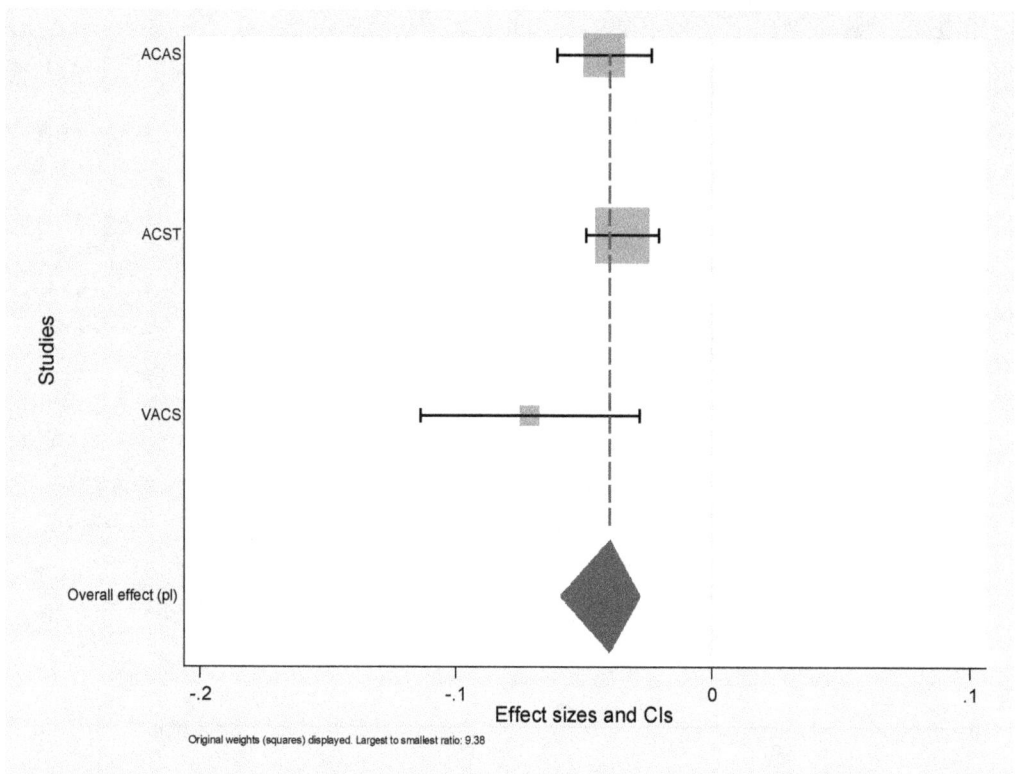

```
--------------------------------------------------------------
   Study      |  Effect  [95% Conf. Interval]  % Weight
--------------+-----------------------------------------------
ACAS          |  -0.042   -0.060    -0.024      34.67
ACST          |  -0.035   -0.049    -0.021      59.04
VACS          |  -0.071   -0.114    -0.028       6.29
--------------+-----------------------------------------------
Overall effect (pl) |  -0.039   -0.058   -0.028   100.00
--------------------------------------------------------------
```

Appendix F Figure 17. Any Stroke (Nonperioperative) for CEA Compared With Medical Therapy, Sensitivity Analysis Using Profile Likelihood Methods

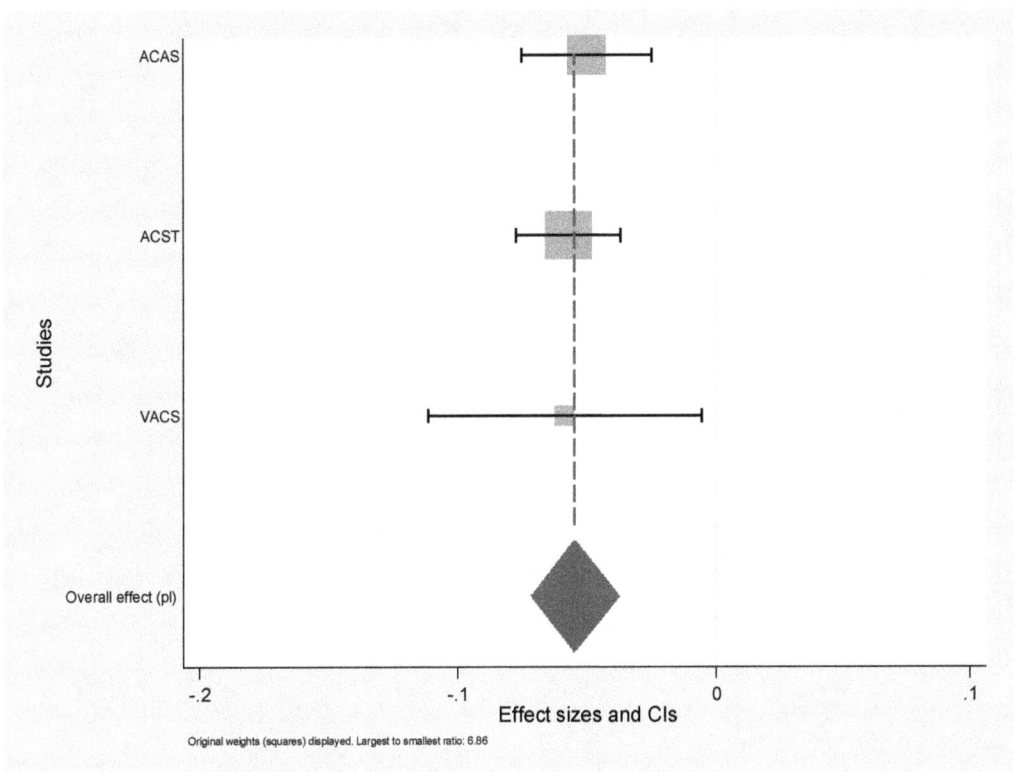

Study		Effect	[95% Conf. Interval]		% Weight
ACAS	|	-0.050	-0.075	-0.025	35.98
ACST	|	-0.057	-0.077	-0.037	55.88
VACS	|	-0.059	-0.111	-0.006	8.14
Overall effect (pl)	|	-0.055	-0.071	-0.038	100.00

Appendix F Figure 18. Perioperative Stroke/Death or Any Subsequent Stroke for CEA Compared With Medical Therapy, Sensitivity Analysis Using Profile Likelihood Methods

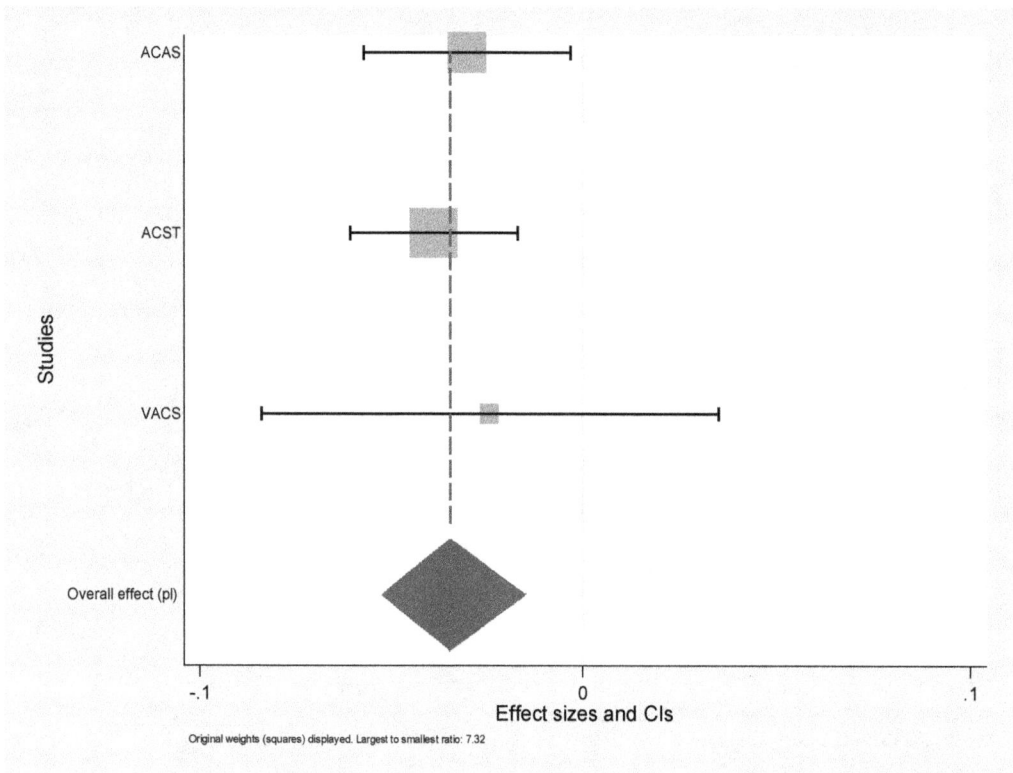

Original weights (squares) displayed. Largest to smallest ratio: 7.32

```
-------------------------------------------------------
  Study    | Effect  [95% Conf. Interval]  % Weight
-----------+-------------------------------------------
ACAS       | -0.030   -0.058   -0.003       36.57
ACST       | -0.039   -0.061   -0.017       55.81
VACS       | -0.024   -0.084    0.035        7.62
-----------+-------------------------------------------
Overall effect (pl) | -0.035  -0.052  -0.015  100.00
-------------------------------------------------------
```

Appendix F Figure 19. Perioperative Stroke/Death or Any Subsequent Stroke for CEA Compared With Medical Therapy, Sensitivity Analysis Including Angiogram-Related Events and Using Profile Likelihood Methods

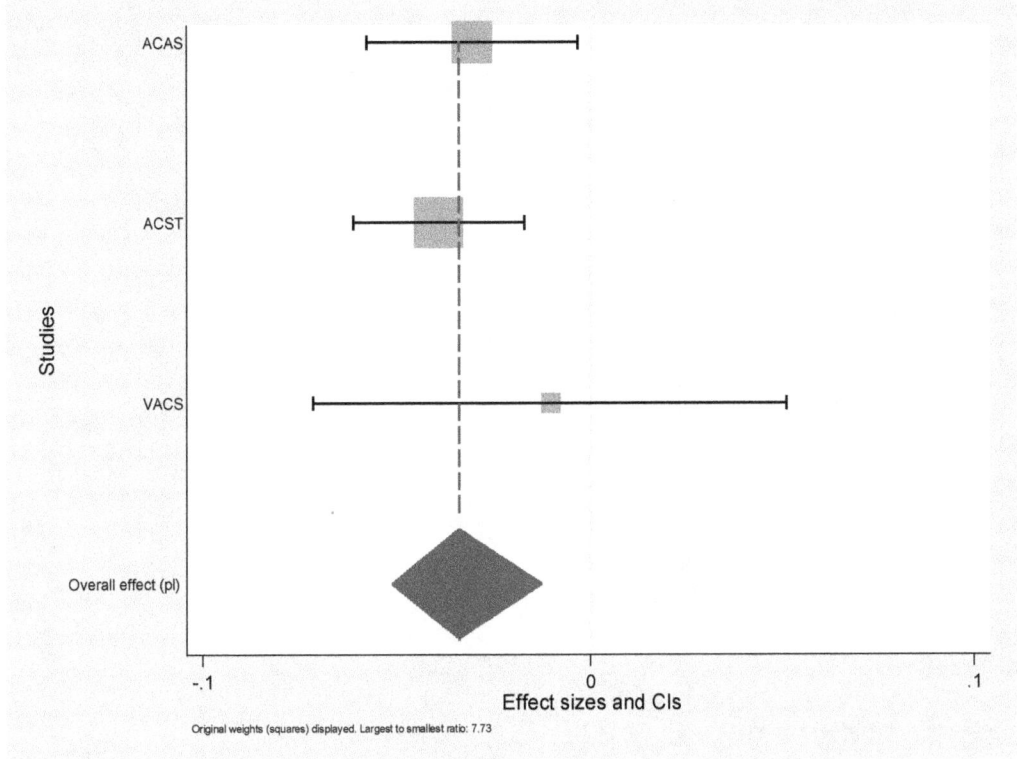

Study	Effect	[95% Conf. Interval]		% Weight
ACAS	-0.030	-0.058	-0.003	36.72
ACST	-0.039	-0.061	-0.017	56.03
VACS	-0.010	-0.072	0.051	7.24
Overall effect (pl)	-0.034	-0.051	-0.013	100.00

Appendix F Figure 20. Perioperative Stroke/Death or Any Subsequent Ipsilateral Stroke for CEA Compared With Medical Therapy, Sensitivity Analysis Using Profile Likelihood Methods

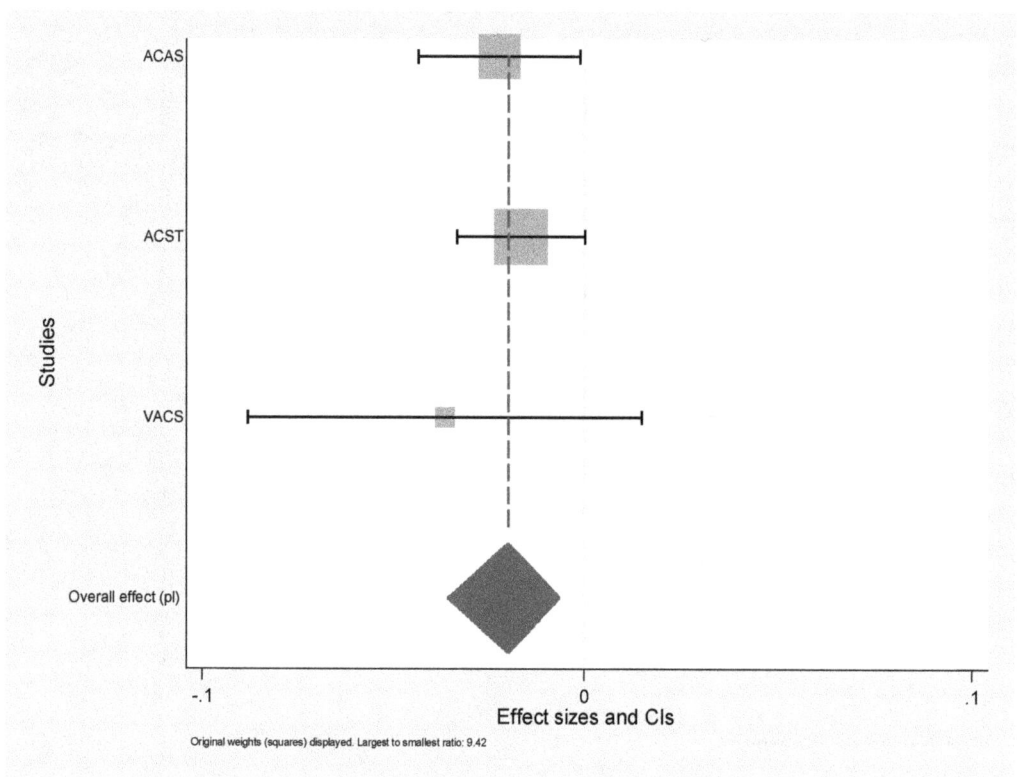

Study	Effect	[95% Conf. Interval]		% Weight
ACAS	-0.022	-0.044	-0.001	36.21
ACST	-0.017	-0.033	0.000	57.67
VACS	-0.037	-0.088	0.015	6.12
Overall effect (pl)	-0.020	-0.036	-0.007	100.00

Appendix F Figure 21. Perioperative Stroke/Death or Any Subsequent Ipsilateral Stroke for CEA Compared With Medical Therapy, Sensitivity Analysis Including Angiogram-Related Events and Using Profile Likelihood Methods

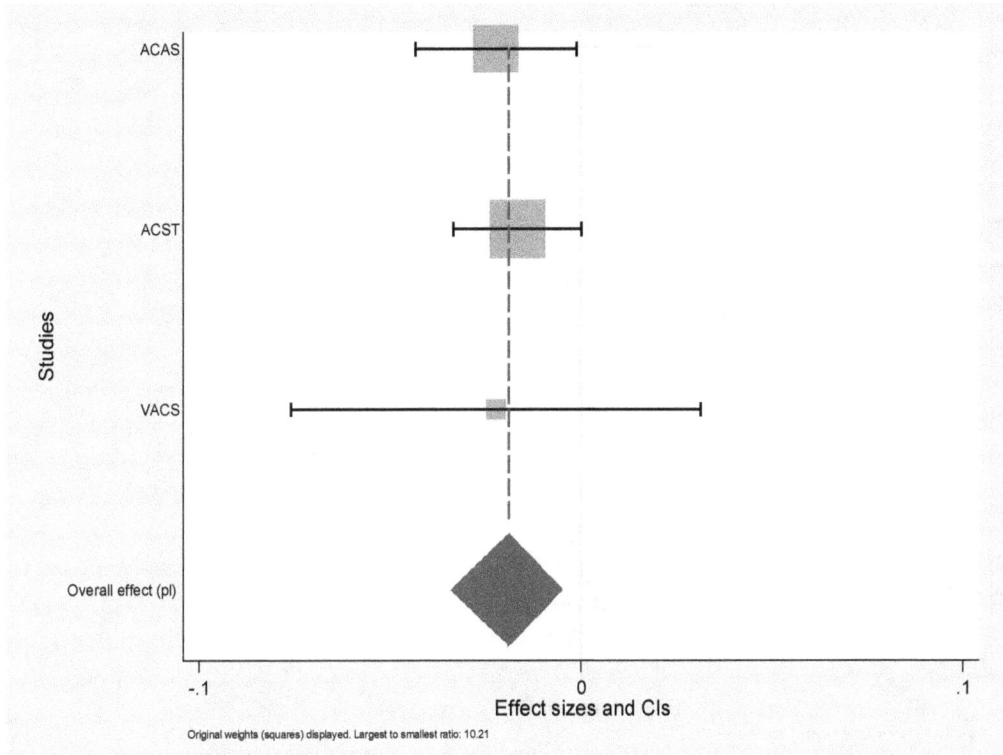

```
--------------------------------------------------------
   Study      | Effect  [95% Conf. Interval]  % Weight
--------------+-----------------------------------------
ACAS          |  -0.022   -0.044   -0.001     36.38
ACST          |  -0.017   -0.033    0.000     57.95
VACS          |  -0.022   -0.076    0.031      5.68
--------------+-----------------------------------------
Overall effect (pl) |  -0.019  -0.034   -0.005   100.00
--------------------------------------------------------
```

Appendix F Figure 22. All-Cause Mortality for CEA Compared With Medical Therapy, Sensitivity Analysis Using Profile Likelihood Methods

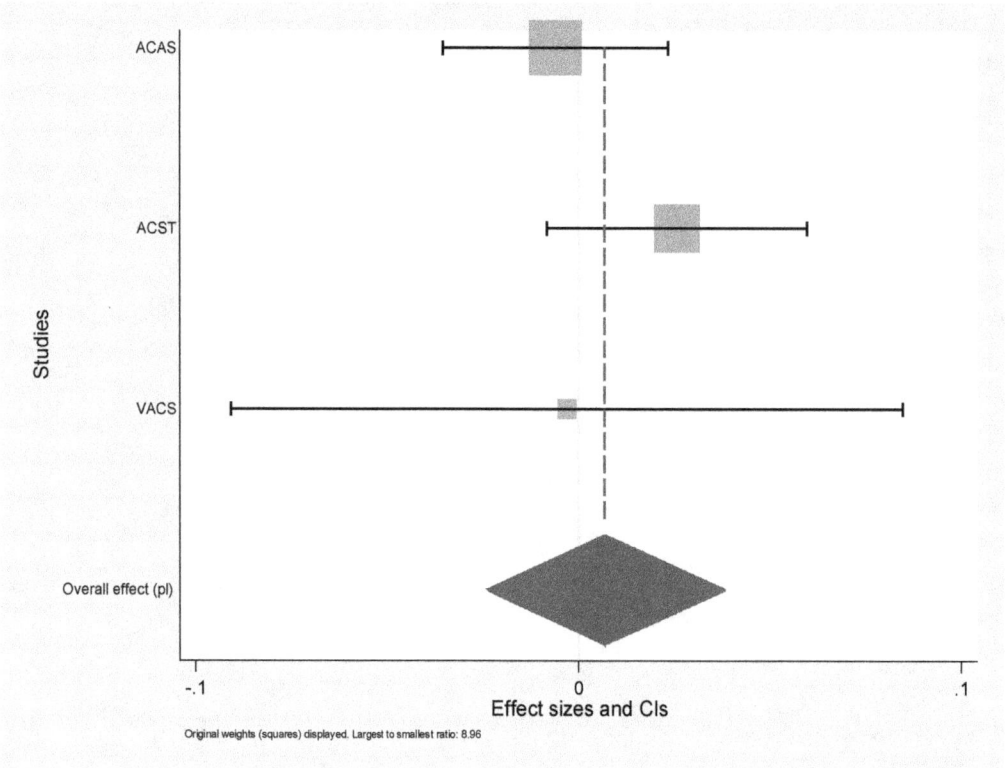

Original weights (squares) displayed. Largest to smallest ratio: 8.96

```
---------------------------------------------------------------
    Study      |  Effect  [95% Conf. Interval]  % Weight
---------------+-----------------------------------------------
ACAS           |  -0.006   -0.035    0.023       53.91
ACST           |   0.026   -0.008    0.060       40.08
VACS           |  -0.003   -0.091    0.085        6.02
---------------+-----------------------------------------------
Overall effect (pl) |  0.007   -0.024    0.038      100.00
---------------------------------------------------------------
```

Appendix F Figure 23. Any Stroke or Death for CEA Compared With Medical Therapy, Sensitivity Analysis Using Profile Likelihood Methods

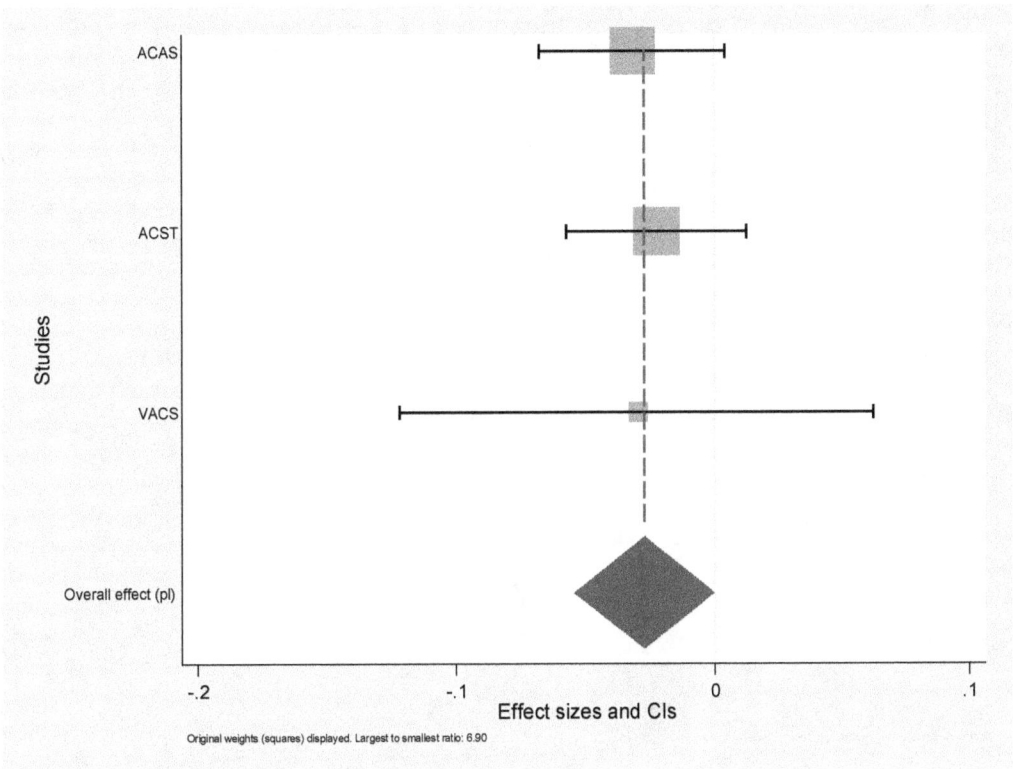

Original weights (squares) displayed. Largest to smallest ratio: 6.90

Study	Effect	[95% Conf. Interval]		% Weight
ACAS	-0.032	-0.068	0.004	45.17
ACST	-0.022	-0.057	0.013	47.89
VACS	-0.030	-0.122	0.062	6.94
Overall effect (pl)	-0.027	-0.054	-0.001	100.00

Appendix F Figure 24. Perioperative Stroke or Death for CEA Compared With Medical Therapy, Sensitivity Analysis Using Profile Likelihood Methods

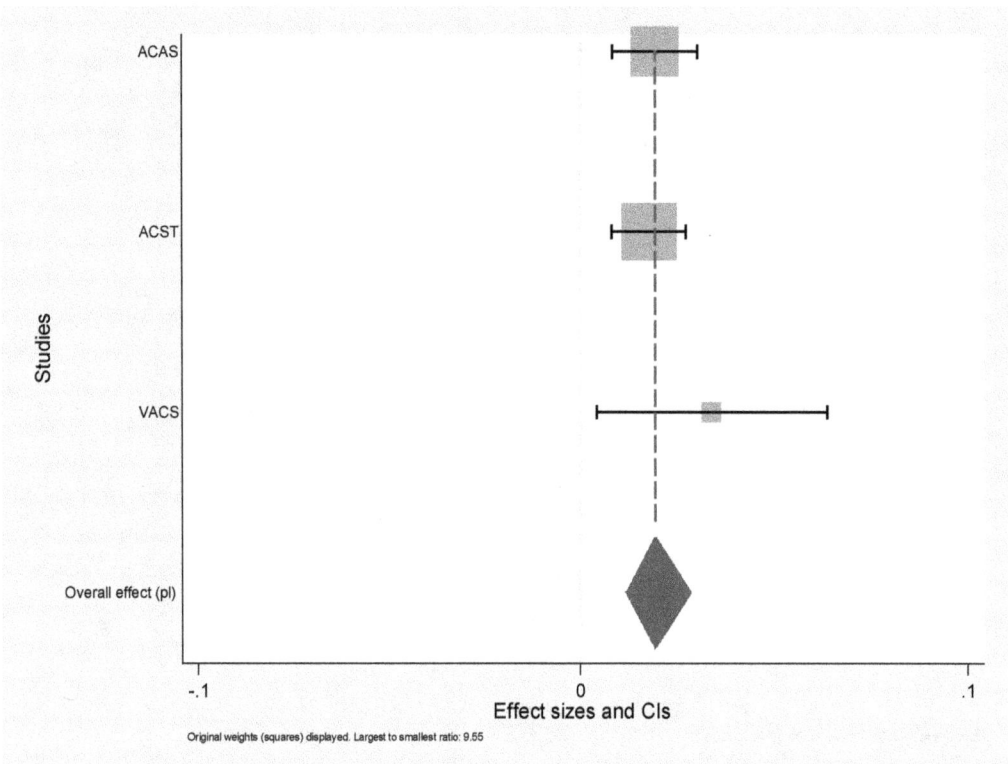

Study		Effect	[95% Conf. Interval]		% Weight
ACAS		0.019	0.008	0.030	40.84
ACST		0.018	0.008	0.028	53.55
VACS		0.034	0.004	0.064	5.60
Overall effect (pl)		0.019	0.012	0.028	100.00

Appendix F Figure 25. Perioperative Stroke or Death for CEA Compared With Medical Therapy, Sensitivity Analysis Including Angiogram-Related Events and Using Profile Likelihood Methods

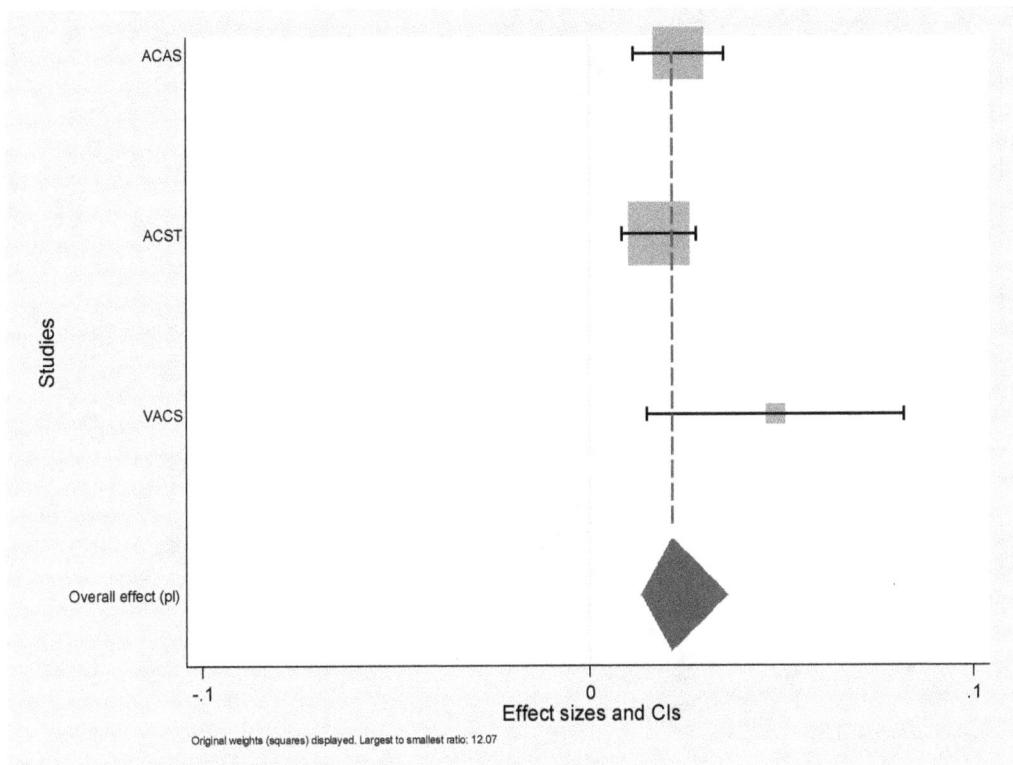

```
--------------------------------------------------------
   Study      | Effect  [95% Conf. Interval]  % Weight
--------------+-----------------------------------------
ACAS          |  0.023   0.011   0.035        38.34
ACST          |  0.018   0.008   0.028        56.94
VACS          |  0.048   0.015   0.082         4.72
--------------+-----------------------------------------
Overall effect (pl) |  0.021   0.014   0.035   100.00
--------------------------------------------------------
```

Appendix F Figure 26. Perioperative Nonfatal Myocardial Infarction for CEA Compared With Medical Therapy, Sensitivity Analysis Using Profile Likelihood Methods

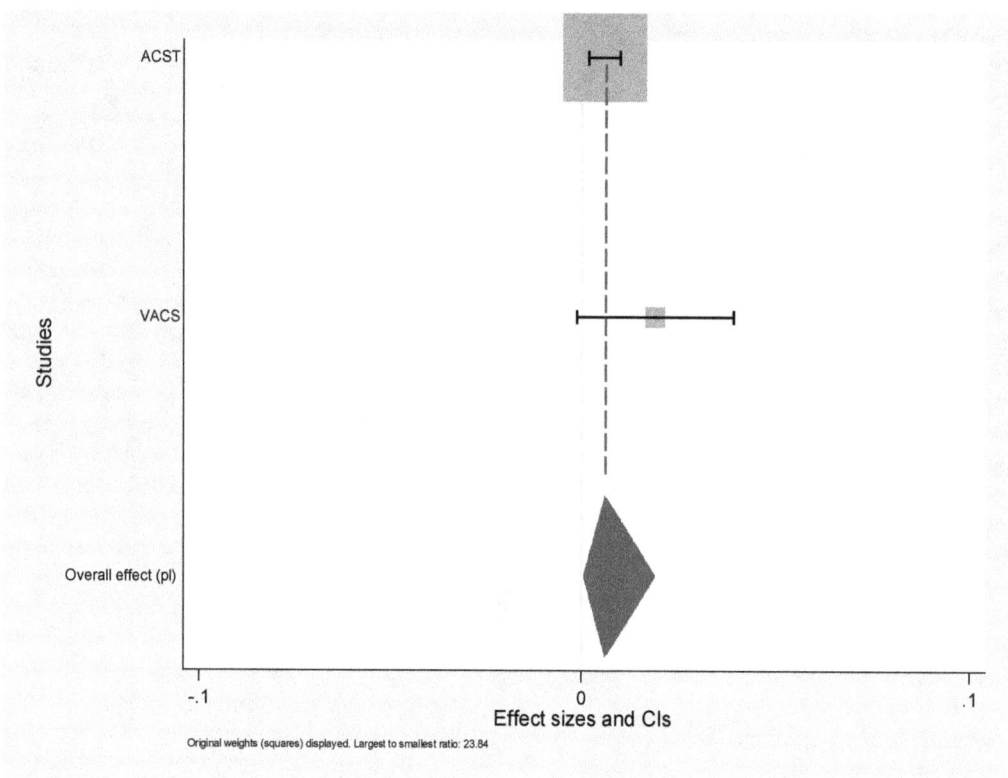

Original weights (squares) displayed. Largest to smallest ratio: 23.84

```
----------------------------------------------------------
   Study      | Effect  [95% Conf. Interval]  % Weight
--------------+-------------------------------------------
ACST          |  0.006   0.002   0.010         95.97
VACS          |  0.019  -0.001   0.039          4.03
--------------+-------------------------------------------
Overall effect (pl) |  0.006   0.001   0.019   100.00
----------------------------------------------------------
```

Appendix F Figure 27. Perioperative Death or Stroke Rate Reported in Trials After CAAS, Sensitivity Analysis Using Profile Likelihood Methods

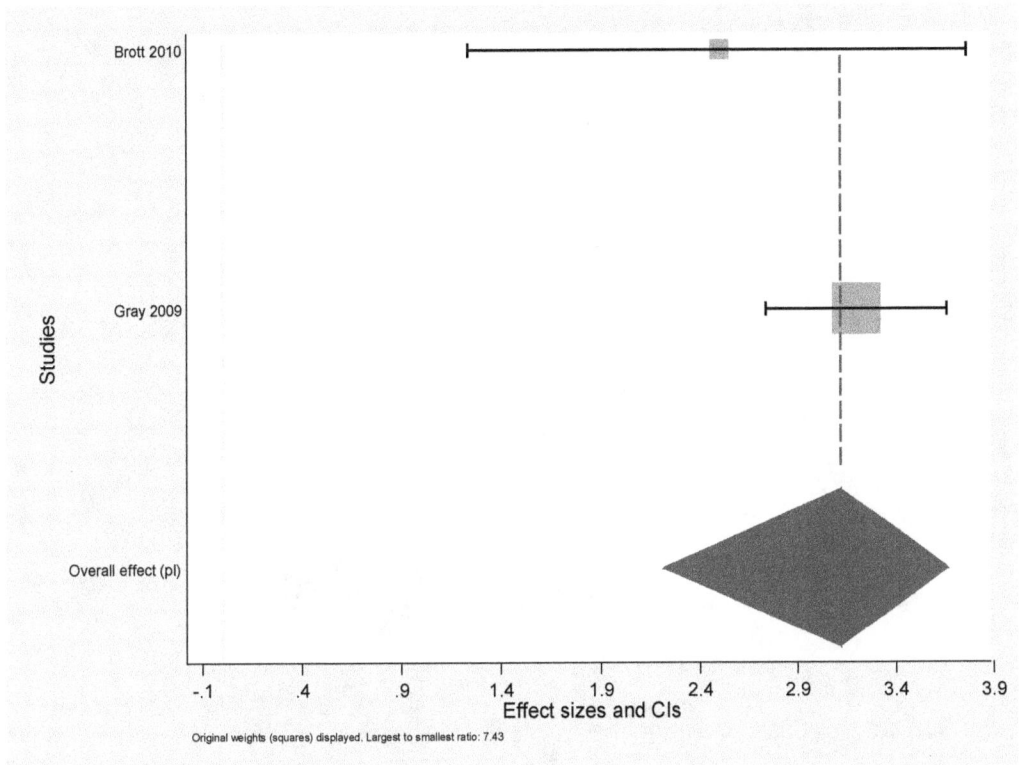

Profile Likelihood method selected

```
--------------------------------------------------------------------
   Study       |  Effect  [95% Conf. Interval]  % Weight
----------------+---------------------------------------------------
Brott 2010      |  2.500    1.238    3.762       11.86
Gray 2009       |  3.200    2.737    3.663       88.14
----------------+---------------------------------------------------
Overall effect (pl) |  3.117   2.224   3.661      100.00
--------------------------------------------------------------------
```

Appendix F Figure 28. Perioperative Death or Stroke Rate Reported in Trials After CAAS, Sensitivity Analysis Using Profile Likelihood Methods and Including Poor Quality Studies

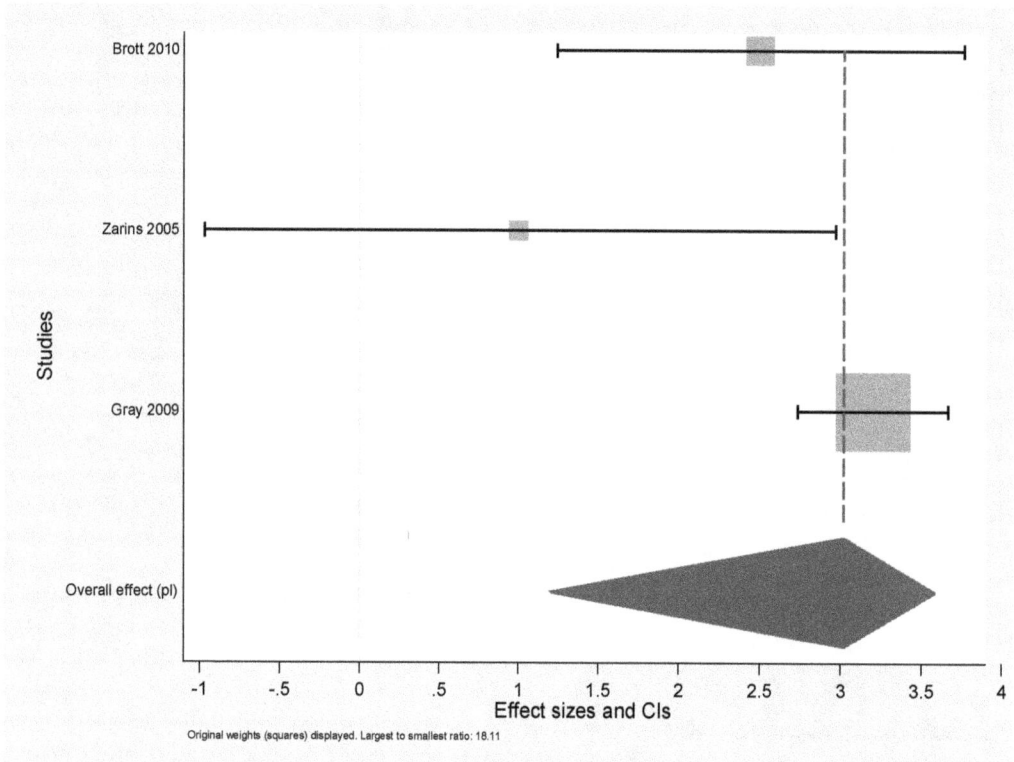

Study	Effect	[95% Conf. Interval]	% Weight
Brott 2010	2.500	1.238	3.762	11.31
Zarins 2005	1.000	-0.970	2.970	4.64
Gray 2009	3.200	2.737	3.663	84.05
Overall effect (pl)	3.019	1.202	3.582	100.00

Appendix F Figure 29. Perioperative Death or Stroke Rate Reported in Cohort Studies After CAAS, Sensitivity Analysis Using Profile Likelihood Methods and Including Poor Quality Studies

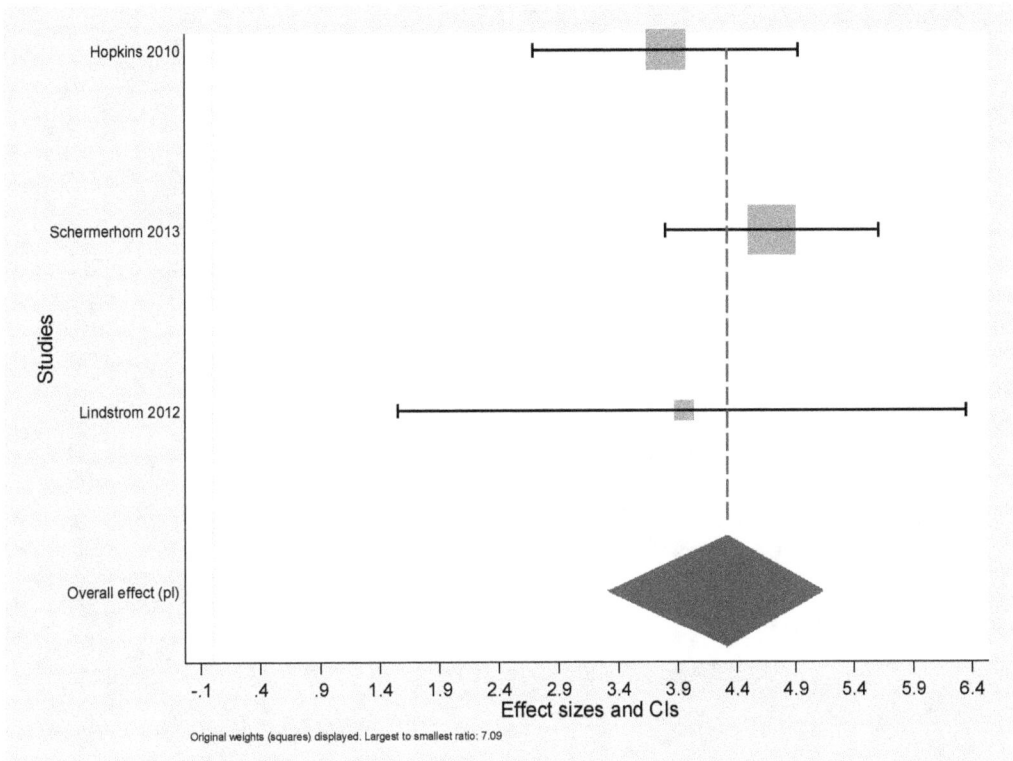

```
--------------------------------------------------------
   Study      |  Effect  [95% Conf. Interval]  % Weight
--------------+-----------------------------------------
Hopkins 2010  |  3.800    2.683    4.917        36.34
Schermerhorn 2013|  4.700    3.798    5.602     55.80
Lindstrom 2012 |  3.952    1.551    6.353        7.87
--------------+-----------------------------------------
Overall effect (pl) |  4.314   3.329   5.115   100.00
--------------------------------------------------------
```

www.ingramcontent.com/pod-product-compliance
Lightning Source LLC
Chambersburg PA
CBHW080639180526
45168CB00008B/3229